The
Multiple Sclerosis
Diet Plan & Cookbook

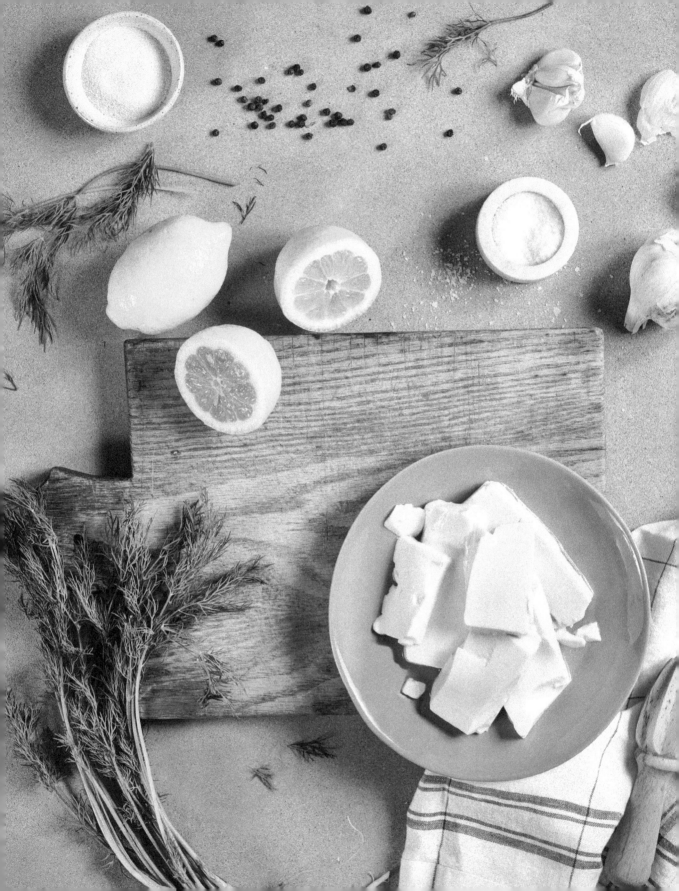

The
Multiple Sclerosis
Diet Plan & Cookbook

101 Easy Anti-Inflammatory Recipes

Noelle DeSantis, MS, RD, CDN

ROCKRIDGE
PRESS

Interior and Cover Designer: Matt Girard
Art Producer: Janice Ackerman
Editor: Michael Goodman
Production Editor: Jenna Dutton

Cover Photography: © 2019 Darren Muir. Food Styling by Yolanda Muir.

Interior Photography: © 2019 Cayla Zahoran. Food styling by Jennifer Ophir. Nadine Greeff: xii; 20; 32; 58; p. 192: Zeynepogan/istock.

ISBN: Print 978-1-64152-871-9 | eBook 978-1-64152-872-6
R0

To Lacey and Sue, two of the most caring and outstanding physical therapists working to improve the lives of those living with MS. And to all the resilient people I have had the pleasure to meet and work with, in research and in practice.

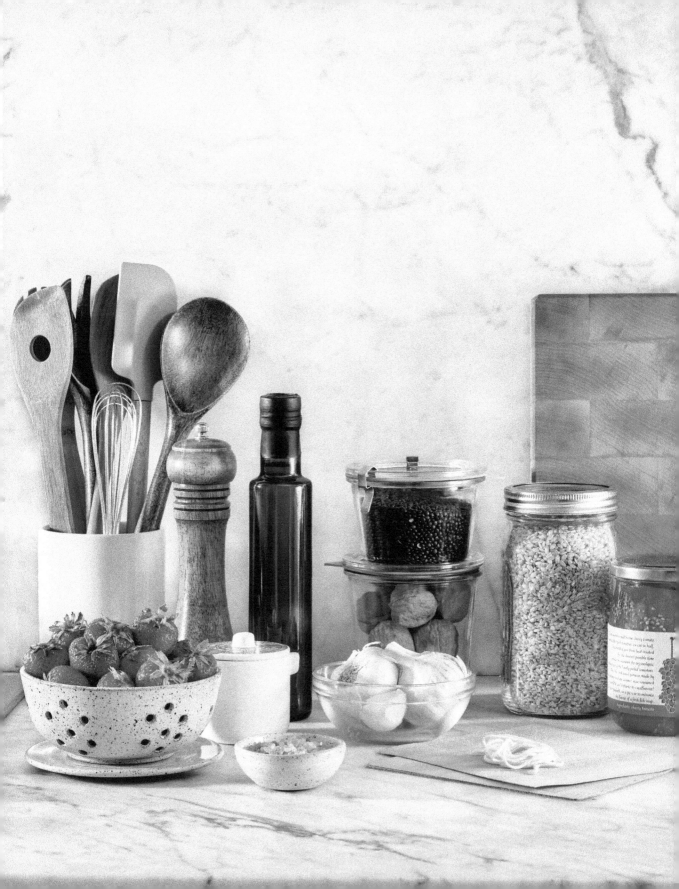

Contents

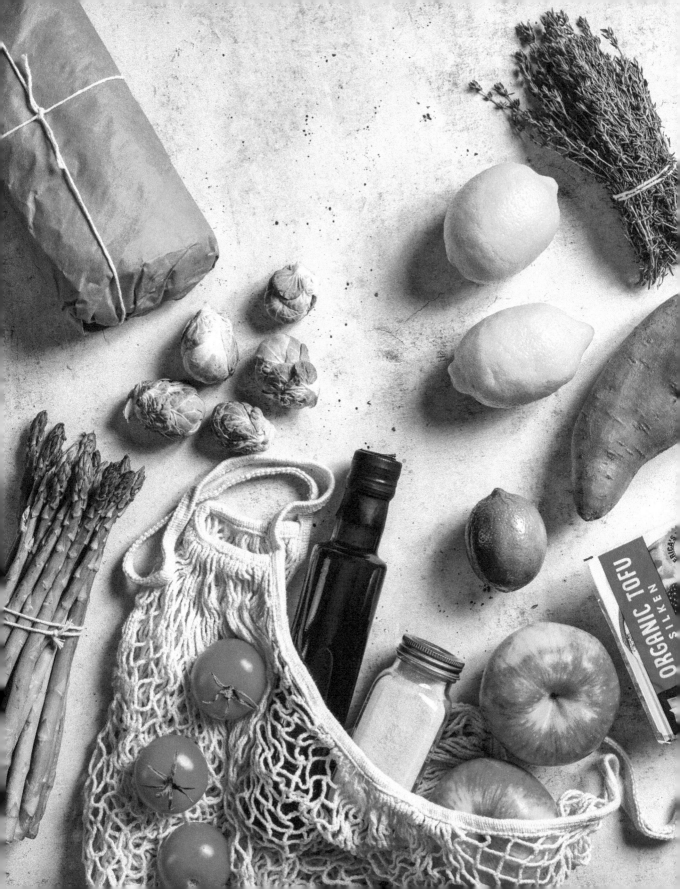

Introduction

Welcome to this anti-inflammatory diet approach to managing multiple sclerosis (MS). Whether you have just started reading about complementary approaches to living well with MS or you've been reading about them for years, I'm glad you're here.

This is not only a diet approach; it's a holistic program to help optimize your quality of life. Whether you have been recently diagnosed or have been living with MS for some time, coming to grips with your body's changes can be difficult. Even thinking about the possibility of changes can be overwhelming.

While multiple sclerosis is not curable, it is manageable and there are steps you can take to keep it as dormant as possible. I have worked with people who have improved some of their symptoms, in addition to preventing flares and further decline. Working in a physical therapy clinic that specializes in neurological conditions allowed me to see some amazing people dedicated to improving their physical abilities as well as their overall quality of life.

This experience solidified my passion for recommending a holistic approach to wellness. A lifestyle that includes physical activity, proper nutrition, and healthy relationships is all part of managing any disease, especially an unpredictable one like MS.

Coping with a debilitating disease is not easy. At times, it may feel frightening, or even impossible, but I want you to know you're not alone. In addition to your friends, family, and health care providers, there are many resilient people who are managing MS with whom you can connect. Approximately one million people in the United States and two million worldwide are living with MS.

In western New York, where I am from, the prevalence of the disease is high, and the diagnosis rate is twice the national average. With a large community of people with MS, there are also many support groups and organizations that offer resources to help those living with the diagnosis. Becoming a member of a support group or participating in a class is a way you can build your resiliency and improve your quality of life.

Each person living with MS is going to have a unique experience. Just remember that, in most cases, those living with MS will have the same longevity as those without it. The key to living well with MS is learning how to manage your symptoms—and how to hone your resiliency.

An array of treatment options now exists, including dietary approaches and disease-modifying medications. Just as no specific medication is best for everyone, there are many dietary approaches as well. I understand that having too many options can lead to uncertainty about how to proceed, but this book follows evidence-based principles. The dietary and lifestyle approaches presented here are realistic, sustainable solutions for managing MS and improving quality of life.

The recommendations in this book promote overall wellness, including emotional, physical, and social health. With easy-to-prepare meals, loaded with anti-inflammatory foods that are not too exotic or pricey, this book is practical for anyone looking to improve wellness and manage symptoms.

My approach to managing MS in clinical practice is more individualized, but the principles in this book will get you started on an anti-inflammatory diet pattern and lifestyle. The anti-inflammatory approach is rich in important nutrients that support brain health, neuroplasticity, and energy production while avoiding foods that may trigger relapse and promote disease progression. The evidence is strong that eating whole foods—mostly nutrient-dense plants—and healthy omega-9 and omega-3 fatty acids, as well as getting adequate hydration, fiber, and protein, is key.

Of course, nutrition, digestion, and absorption are the primary lifestyle factors I want to optimize, but there is so much more. Behavior change is another big component. Even something that sounds as trivial as how quickly you eat your food can have an impact on digestion and gastrointestinal symptoms.

I promote a holistic approach, so I consider the whole person. This includes environment, stress, sleep patterns, and bowel and urinary health, as well as nutrient status and hormones. Emotions and relationships are also an important part of wellness—having healthy relationships with others and yourself is crucial.

This book will offer you tips for managing stress, improving the quality of your sleep, slowing down at the table, and choosing foods that support brain and immune health while decreasing inflammation. These delicious, anti-inflammatory dishes are healthy for the whole family and won't require making separate meals for individual family members.

I also include tips and substitution suggestions for food intolerances, shortcuts, and allergies. (For example, using pumpkin seeds in place of a tree nut can keep the crunch and the healthy fats in a dish while removing an allergen.) In addition to recipes, you will find other helpful advice, such as how to make meal preparation easier and modified-utensil recommendations.

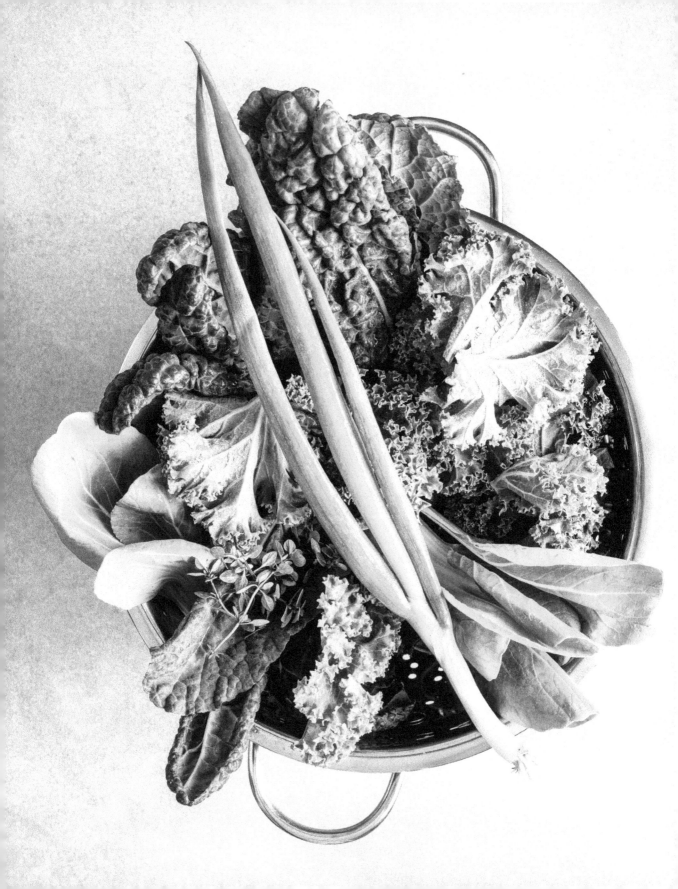

PART ONE

Before You Begin

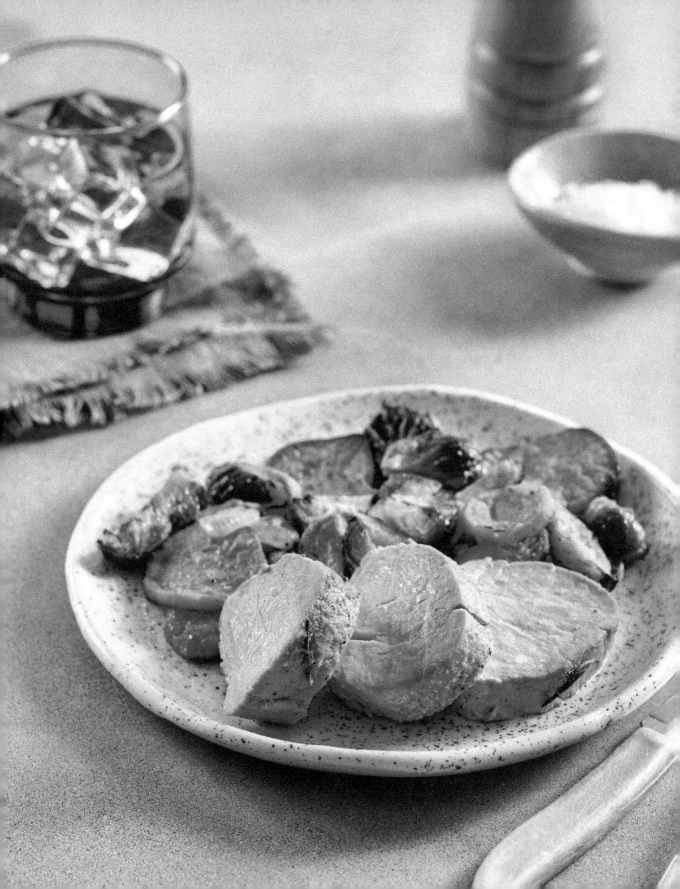

CHAPTER ONE

Where Diet Intersects Well-Being

I am so excited you have decided to embark on this journey and take actionable steps to manage your MS symptoms and prevent flares to improve your quality of life. With a wealth of information available online, it can be daunting to decide which approach is best for you. As a registered dietitian with a passion for helping individuals with MS improve their overall wellness, I have put together an easy-to-follow plan to help make your journey smoother and more enjoyable.

In this chapter, I will offer a few tips, outline how diet can influence disease outcomes, and explore some popular diet approaches. I will also briefly explain the gut-brain connection and the gut-immune connection (my favorite thing to talk about).

What Brought You Here?

Think about why you've come to this book. Maybe your best friend has been diagnosed and you are learning more about how to support them. Perhaps you are the one newly diagnosed and want to learn more about how lifestyle can impact your disease outcomes. Or it could be that you have been following a specific diet but you feel it's not working.

Are you taking care of someone who has MS and feel that they can improve their quality of life by developing new habits? Do you have specific questions, or are you just looking to learn something new? Maybe you are motivated by something you heard, or you're looking for motivation here.

Whatever it is that brought you to this book, I encourage you to be hopeful about taking these actionable steps. You should look forward to the benefits to your well-being that result from following an anti-inflammatory lifestyle.

You can also use this moment of reflection as an opportunity to record your thoughts or feelings—jot them down in a journal, on your computer, or even in the notes section of your cell phone. You can compare how you feel now to how you are feeling in the future after taking the steps highlighted in this book.

A Simple Approach to a Complex Condition

Making dietary changes can seem difficult, but it doesn't have to be overly complicated—or even boring. It can be fun and delicious. You may have preconceived notions that a "diet" is going to mean too much restriction, no more socializing with friends, and the end of enjoying food. This is simply not the case. It may just mean a little reprogramming of what you think of as an appropriate portion size for protein or how many servings of vegetables and fruit are adequate.

Your own cultural and flavor preferences will remain central—you may just need to modify things you are already doing. I like to use "SMART" (specific, measurable, attainable, relevant, and timely) goals, working on one change at a time, as this results in more-sustainable changes. As MS is an inflammatory disease of the central nervous system, a well-balanced, anti-inflammatory diet rich in brain-supporting nutrients is ideal for managing it.

Consider the possible benefits:

Feel Better

Following a healthy diet pattern will lead to improved overall health and can help alleviate some of the more difficult symptoms you may experience. For example, including adequate fiber, which can improve neurotransmitter production, can boost your mood. It can also improve symptoms related to bowel function. Adequate calories and protein can help keep your energy levels stable and maintain muscle mass.

Improve Outcomes

In general, life expectancy and health outcomes will vary among those with MS. Some specific ways diet can improve outcomes include managing blood sugar, preserving kidney function, supporting joint health, decreasing pain, and preserving lean body mass. Diet can also improve energy, which can help you get through a physical therapy or gym session or a family vacation when you are feeling fatigued.

Build Good Habits

Building good habits is essential to a healthy lifestyle, allowing you to improve or maintain your health almost effortlessly. Remember: Habits are not formed overnight. It takes time to reroute the pathways in your brain to allow you to do things without thinking too much, so try not to get frustrated.

Change Your Outlook

Living with an unpredictable, debilitating disease is not easy, and it's okay to have negative thoughts or a solemn mind-set at times. Trying to change your outlook to be more positive may feel impossible, but once you start to feel better physically, you can begin to feel better mentally, too. Remember: Diet and exercise can improve mood and energy levels, as well as help you get to a positive outlook.

Understanding MS

While disease-modifying drug therapies are advancing, there is still no cure for MS and MS-related symptoms, but an anti-inflammatory diet can be a great complementary or alternative treatment option. There are vast resources available online, as well as MS organizations that can be very helpful for learning more about the disease. In this book, I'm focusing on how diet can impact MS—this is something you can act upon, giving you the power to improve your quality of life.

MS, Briefly

MS is a progressive, immune-mediated, chronic, inflammatory disease of the central nervous system. This means it affects the brain and spinal cord, which you can think of as the body's control center. About 2.3 million people are living with MS worldwide, making it the most common disease of the nervous system. It usually begins between the ages of 20 and 40, and women are more frequently diagnosed than men. Several risk factors have been associated with MS, including:

- Immune dysregulation
- Genetics
- Exposure to the Epstein-Barr virus
- Smoking
- Living in the northern latitudes
- Low vitamin D status
- Diet
- Childhood obesity

In MS, the immune cells that normally protect us by fighting off pathogens and other foreign invaders mistakenly attack myelin, the fatty material that covers our nerve fibers and helps nerve signals travel throughout the body. This results in chronic inflammation in the central nervous system, which eventually leads to demyelination of nerve fibers. When the myelin is lost, nerve transmission is decreased, and, eventually, the underlying nerve fiber is damaged. This damage is seen as lesions in the brain. The disruption of nerve transduction is what ultimately leads to the symptoms of MS: Cells are no longer sending signals required for various functions.

Although MS has no cure (yet), it is manageable. The key to long-term success is preventing flare-ups by decreasing inflammation and exposure to triggers that may ramp up your immune response. You also want to include functional foods that support brain health.

Typical Treatment Options

Many drug therapies are available to modify the course of the disease by targeting immune-cell proliferation and differentiation. This means they target production of immune cells, increasing immune cells that fight inflammation (anti-inflammatory) and decreasing types that ramp up inflammation (pro-inflammatory). These treatments do not cure MS, and they don't come without side effects. Common side effects include injection-site irritation, flu-like symptoms, altered liver function, increased risk of infection, and gastrointestinal symptoms.

Diet is a cost-effective, alternative treatment approach to manage MS symptoms and disease progression. A modified diet can improve outcomes and potentially reduce the dosage and side effects of drug therapies.

Outcomes

MS is an unpredictable disease with outcomes that vary greatly. There are different types of MS and different symptoms depending on which part of the nervous system is affected. The rate of progression and severity of symptoms varies from person to person. I have met people who had one flare and never experienced another symptom, while others have symptoms that progress rapidly. Some of these symptoms may include fatigue, depression, walking difficulties, sleep disturbances, decreased gut motility, and impaired vision. Some of the earliest symptoms are numbness and tingling in extremities, but the most common symptom is fatigue. Many people describe fatigue as the most debilitating issue, since it diminishes their ability to carry out daily activities.

No matter which symptoms you have or what stage the disease has reached, you can take action by choosing an anti-inflammatory diet that can halt or slow the disease's progression. Dietary changes that support a healthy immune system, healthy gastrointestinal tract, and the repair and regrowth of central nervous system tissue will set you up to manage MS successfully.

The recipes in this book keep physical limitations and fatigue in mind. I include foods that support energy production and brain health and fight inflammation to improve your quality of life—and keep MS as dormant as possible.

MS TYPES AND STAGES

The International Advisory Committee on Clinical Trials of Multiple Sclerosis has identified four types of MS, each based on disease activity and progression.

> **Clinically isolated syndrome.** This is a single attack of inflammation and/or demyelination in the central nervous system. At this point, there is no diagnosis of MS, and, in fact, the disease may never develop. It is the first episode of neurological symptoms that are typical of MS. These symptoms may or may not be accompanied by MS-like lesions.

> **Relapsing-remitting.** This is the most common form of MS, presenting in about 80 percent of the disease's population. It's characterized by acute episodes of neurological dysfunction with full or partial recovery. In most people, it usually advances to secondary-progressive MS in 15 to 20 years. Because of the unpredictable nature of the disease, some people may not experience new symptoms or disability following a relapse, while others do. Some will experience progressive disability over time.

> **Secondary-progressive.** This is the second, advanced stage of relapsing-remitting, characterized by progressive disability over time. There may be relapses of inflammation, but there is increasing nerve damage or loss. This MS type has different subtypes based on what is happening at any given time: active (indicates relapse and/or new MRI activity), nonactive (no relapse/activity), with progression (evidence of disease progression), and without progression.

> **Primary-progressive.** This type is characterized by worsening neurological symptoms from the first episode. There is no relapse or remission following progression. The activity here is similar to secondary-progressive activity but without the early stages of relapsing-remitting.

Working Through Your Diagnosis

An MS diagnosis can raise a lot of feelings, not only for the individual but also for friends and family. It is important to focus on your emotional and social wellness in addition to your physical well-being. Engaging your emotions, learning to live in the present, and having realistic expectations are all ways you can work on your emotional health.

Engaging Your Emotions

No matter what you are feeling, know that it is completely valid. Your feelings may not all be positive vibes, sunflowers, and daisies, but they are yours, so try not to suppress them. It's okay to feel angry, sad, confused, or frustrated—trying to avoid those negative feelings can make things worse.

There are many strategies for dealing with overwhelming emotions, and you may need to try a few before you find one that works well for you. Calling a friend, family member, or health care provider can be one place to start. It might also be a good idea to join a support group to become more comfortable talking about your feelings and learn ways to deal with them. You may also try meditation to redirect your thoughts in the moment and practice positive self-talk regularly.

Living in the Present

Life is happening now, all around you. If you are consumed with the past or worrying about the prospects of the future, you may miss out on the beauties and joys of life. I encourage you to slow down and take time to be present. When you feel like your thoughts are overwhelming and encroaching on your present moment, remember to breathe—and then remember that they are just thoughts, and they can be redirected.

This may sound easy, but it will take practice. You first need to recognize that your thoughts are interfering with the present moment, and then you can try to redirect them. A simple meditation can help with this. You can try the meditation I outline later in this book, or you could explore the Internet or your local library for other ideas.

Realistic Expectations

Try to be patient as you move ahead with this diet plan or any other treatment options you may try. Just as forming a new habit takes time, feeling or seeing progress in symptom management and emotional well-being doesn't happen immediately. While some people say they have reversed their disease through diet and lifestyle, they also may have been working on perfecting their bio-individuality for years.

Reversing every symptom may not be a realistic goal, but enhancing your quality of life can be. I have worked with people who have significantly improved their physical abilities, but it took dedication and commitment to diet and physical activity over a period of time.

Patience will be key to keeping you on track—and keeping you from becoming discouraged. I want you to know that committing to anti-inflammatory lifestyle changes can help you manage your disease and symptoms. Managing the disease can significantly improve your quality of life.

A Shift to Diet

There is not a specific diet recommended for individuals living with MS, partly due to the lack of clinical control trials (considered the gold standard for research). Few clinical trials have looked at the effects of dietary intervention on disease progression. Over the years, many approaches have been recommended that seem to have some benefits for MS. You may have heard of and even tried some of these diets.

Swank (low-fat)

This is one of the oldest diet approaches for managing MS, developed by Dr. Roy Swank in the 1950s after his observational findings linked increased saturated-fat intake to a higher prevalence of MS. The Swank diet limits saturated fat to 15 grams per day and unsaturated fat to 20 to 50 grams per day. It also encourages whole grains, fish in any amount, low-fat dairy, trimmed poultry, and a limit of 3 ounces of red meat per week.

The report that followed 144 patients on the diet for 70 years concluded that a strict low-fat diet can improve disease survival, ambulation, and overall outcomes. This study was observational and had no control group. Also, there was no measure of fatigue severity despite reporting that participants were very active and able to care for themselves at follow-up.

Wahls (modified Paleo)

Dr. Terry Wahls developed the Wahls Protocol, based on a modified Paleolithic diet, after she explored Paleo and functional medicine to help manage her own MS. She reported that this lifestyle change helped dramatically improve her quality of life—and even reversed her disease progression.

The principles of the Paleo diet call for whole, unprocessed foods with a low-glycemic index, game meat, organ meat, wild fish, and nine daily servings of fruits and vegetables. It excludes dairy, eggs, and gluten (gluten-free grains and legumes are limited to two servings per week). Seaweed and fermented foods are also recommended.

The premise is that you can get adequate nutrients from the variety of fruits and vegetables, organ meat, and other recommended foods and supplements, while also optimizing mitochondrial function and energy by reaching ketosis (see "Other Options" on page 13). When eliminating entire food groups, it's important to make sure that your calorie needs are met and you're getting enough vitamin D.

Boroch (candida-free)

This approach was developed by Ann Boroch following her own diagnosis of MS, after which she remained symptom-free for 23 years. The diet involves eliminating alcohol, sugar, corn, caffeine, dairy, gluten, soy, fermented foods, and fruits, with the exceptions of berries, green apples, grapefruit, avocado, lemon, lime, and olives without vinegar brine. The premise is that poor diet, stress, heavy metals, and alcohol intake inhibit the proliferation of good bacteria in the gut, allowing candida to overgrow.

Candida is a harmless yeast found on the skin and in the gut of every healthy person. The problem is that when it overgrows, it causes an imbalance in our microbiome. By eliminating the foods that candida can thrive on (sugars, refined carbohydrates, dairy, and other processed foods), you can reduce the candida and restore balance in the gut.

Regular bowel movements are encouraged, along with supplements like flax-seed to aid them, if necessary. This diet is meant to be short-term (90 days) and followed according to the 80/20 rule: 80 percent of the time you avoid the foods candida thrives on, and 20 percent of the time you can treat yourself to a glass of wine, a slice of pizza, or a piece of cake. Once the candida level is brought into balance, you can enjoy yeast-promoting foods in moderation. The evidence for this approach comes mainly from case studies.

Putting It All Together

The anti-inflammatory diet in this book is a plant-forward approach with whole foods at the center. You can customize it according to your unique needs and preferences. Limiting saturated fat is important because saturated and trans fats are pro-inflammatory. But that doesn't mean this diet is low-fat—omega-9 and omega-3 fatty acids are anti-inflammatory, and their food sources are often also a great source of fiber, which is fuel for the bacteria in the gut that play a key role in immune and overall health.

The basics of the diet include filling your plate with a variety of colorful fruits and vegetables rich in anti-inflammatory and essential nutrients, varied protein sources, and healthy fats to complement the meals. Foods to avoid include highly processed foods, deep-fried foods, and foods that contain allergens or cause intolerance. Things to limit include sugar, sodium, and alcohol.

Other important aspects of this holistic approach include portion control, adequate hydration, regenerative and restful sleep, physical activity, and mindfulness.

OTHER OPTIONS

In addition to specific food recommendations, there are some additional diet approaches you might consider, including ketosis, intermittent fasting, and extended overnight fasting.

Ketosis is the state that describes using fat as your primary source of fuel instead of carbohydrates. It requires carbohydrate restriction to between 20 and 50 grams per day, causing your body to switch to using the ketones from fat as fuel instead of the glucose from carbs. It is a very restrictive approach—you have to really limit all carbs including fruits and starchy vegetables. Speak to a health care provider before starting this strategy, especially if you take glucose-lowering medications or have kidney disease.

Some evidence exists that intermittent fasting can change gut bacteria and reduce inflammation in people with MS by fasting two days per week. During fasting days, you restrict yourself to 500 calories per day. Experimental studies have shown immune modulation, changes in hormones, neuroprotection, and increased microbial diversity from intermittent fasting. However, the feasibility and effects of long-term practice are not known and are currently being investigated.

An alternative form of fasting is extended overnight fasting. This can be achieved by having your last meal three hours before bed and then fasting eight hours while you sleep plus an additional hour or two after waking. This may not be for everyone—a healthy snack before bed may be beneficial depending on your health conditions.

This book is not meant to stand in for medical treatment. Make sure you consult your primary health care provider before starting this diet or any of the diet approaches mentioned previously.

The Gut-Brain Connection

There is growing evidence that the gut microbiome can have a large impact on neurodegenerative diseases. You may have heard of the gut-brain axis or heard the gut referred to as the "second brain." A large part of this is related to the gut microbiome.

Your Microbiome

The gastrointestinal tract is home to trillions of microorganisms, mainly bacteria that make up the gut microbiome. A number of things can contribute to the makeup of your gut microbiome, diet being the main influencer.

Three main types of microorganisms exist in the gut. First are symbionts, which promote health by maintaining gut integrity, producing vitamins and neurotransmitters, protecting against pathogens, and regulating immunity. Next are commensals, which appear to have no direct effect on health. Last are pathobionts, which can cause inflammation. Research shows that the microorganisms in our gut communicate in a bidirectional manner with our central nervous system, immune cells, and endocrine system. This communication contributes to the gut-brain axis.

Neurotransmitters

These chemical messengers help our neurons (the cells in the central nervous system) communicate with each other and, in turn, communicate with every system in the body. Our microbiota not only stimulate production of neurotransmitters in the gut, they also produce several other neurotransmitters. These include serotonin, dopamine, norepinephrine, and gamma-aminobutyric acid. It is estimated that 80 to 90 percent of the body's serotonin is produced in the gut. This is incredible, as these neurotransmitters help regulate mood, sleep, appetite, pain perception, and digestion.

Axis of Inflammation

The microorganisms in the gut also talk with immune cells. By-products of bacterial cells that favor fermentation of plant foods produce important short-chain fatty acids. Some of these fatty acids promote healing in the gut and stimulate proteins at tight junctions. This protects the integrity of the gastro-intestinal tract, which serves as the first line of defense against inflammation in the gut. The metabolites produced by certain symbiotic microbes actually inhibit pro-inflammatory immune cells and promote anti-inflammatory immune cells. Tryptophan is also metabolized by the microbiome, producing aryl hydrocarbon receptor (AhR) ligands, which reduce inflammation in the central nervous system.

On the other hand, a diet that is high in added sugars, sodium, and animal fat and low in fiber results in different by-products that break down intestinal-cell-wall integrity.

Why It Matters

The standard American diet (high in animal fat, sodium, and sugar and low in fiber) results in an increase in inflammatory cells and the endotoxin lipopoly-saccharide, leading to a chain reaction of increased circulating inflammatory cytokines. Paired with the breakdown of the gut cell wall, this leads to systemic inflammation, meaning the inflammation can now enter the bloodstream. This can cause increased blood-brain-barrier permeability and inflammation in the central nervous system. A healthy diet rich in fruits, vegetables, whole grains, nuts, seeds, and healthy fat will promote a diverse microbiome that can influence immune response. A healthy microbiome can improve MS symptoms and slow progression.

A Three-Pronged Approach

Managing MS requires you to consider more than diet alone. In this book, I will focus on proper nutrition, your lifestyle, and your support team.

Diet

Changing your diet will help improve physical well-being in a number of ways. As I previously mentioned, your diet can influence your microbiome, which impacts immune health and cognitive health. Balance in neurotransmitter production can improve your mood and motivation and help with energy and pain. Having adequate fiber in your diet will support those functions of the healthy microbiome. Phytonutrients (the compounds responsible for a plant food's color, scent, and taste) are anti-inflammatory and can help promote brain and heart health and protect against cancer.

Lifestyle

Taking care of your body and mind is just as important as optimizing dietary intake. You may be eating all the healthy foods recommended, but physical activity is necessary as well. Physical activity can help maintain lean body mass and promote heart health and is an opportunity for cortical reorganization and neural repair. A 2017 review published in the journal *Neural Plasticity* looked at the role of exercise in increasing the production of neurotrophins, which play a role in neuronal repair and plasticity. The review concluded that prescribed exercise could improve wellness, reduce symptoms, and reduce inflammation.

Your Team

Your support team is equally important in this three-pronged approach. You want people on your side who are supporting your efforts to improve your health and overall wellness. It may not always be easy to get loved ones or friends on board with your lifestyle changes, so educating them on how the changes can help you is important. The great thing about this approach is that it will promote healthly choices for anyone who makes the changes with you.

Your health care providers are important, too, so make sure you are comfortable with the providers you choose and that you talk with them about anything you are experiencing.

What to Expect

This book is meant to be a helpful, informational guide to get you started on a holistic approach to managing MS. If you want to learn more about anything you've read so far, I recommend diving deeper into the research, especially information on the gut-brain axis and immune modulation, as well as the benefits of exercise and mind-body techniques.

In the next chapter, you will find the beginning of your process, starting with a commitment. You will also find simple, actionable steps regarding physical activity and mindfulness. I strongly encourage you to modify these, add to them, and work on them with your support team and/or health care providers. Build on your baseline goals, whatever they may be. Spend as much time as you need on your goals before you move on.

Get Your Ducks in a Row

Getting organized for the lifestyle changes you are going to make will help you succeed and stick to the plan. This includes some of the steps in the following chapters, like the pantry clean-out and how to restock. You may find it helpful to make lists or put notes on your calendar. You will also want to explore options for how to build your support team and who the members might be. Don't forget that, as a member of a group, you may be someone else's support teammate, too.

Lifestyle Solutions

Part of making lifestyle changes is planning how they will take place. Who will help? When will they occur? What will you work on first? Where will the behavior take place?

Decide when you are most likely to engage in physical activity, and factor in when you usually have the most energy. If you are planning to practice mindfulness with a friend, make sure to set a date. Habits are not easy to form, so coming up with the best plan is imperative. This may include writing notes to yourself or setting alarms on your phone or in your home for reminders. A friend or family member can be a great motivator, too.

Meal Plan

The bulk of the book is the meal plan, which you will find in the following chapters. It's laid out in an easy-to-follow format, with recipes and pantry staples. The plan includes breakfasts, lunches, dinners, and snacks, as well as grocery lists. This should help alleviate some of the stress around meal planning.

The meal plan has been consciously designed to include variety, with foods that are appealing to the whole family. If you live alone, there are storage tips to help you use the recipes as an opportunity for meal prep. This will save you energy on another day to do something else you enjoy.

Recipes

The recipes are tasty and satisfying without being overly restrictive and include easy-to-find ingredients that can fit into a limited budget. A good variety of cuisines, flavors, and textures is included, keeping the fun and adventure in enjoying a meal.

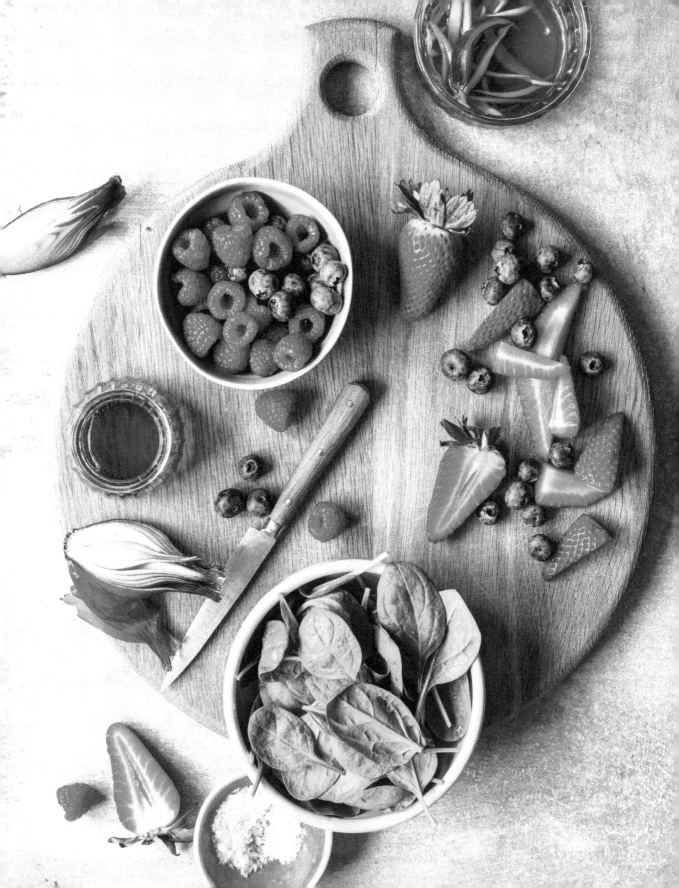

CHAPTER TWO

Getting Ready

Now that you have reflected on what brought you here and learned more about this anti-inflammatory approach, I want to help prepare you for the next steps. This isn't a strict diet plan to immediately dive into—it's a lifestyle, which requires sustainable behavior change. The process will look different for each person. Everyone reading this book has a unique lifestyle and health history. You may have food allergies, previous surgeries, or other health conditions that may require extra fine-tuning with the help of a registered dietitian or health care provider.

You will move through this process at your own pace. In my experience, sustainable behavior change doesn't happen overnight. Small steps toward the ultimate goal are the key to success. Here are the strategies to help you start making changes and feeling better.

Step 1: Make the Commitment

Commit to giving the anti-inflammatory diet approach a try because you believe you can and you know it will improve your quality of life. This is an exciting moment because you are choosing to take control. While you can't control everything in your life, diet and lifestyle are modifiable factors that can help you manage symptoms of MS and prevent relapse and progression.

Building relationships with others who support what you are trying to do will help you make a commitment and stick to it. There is no such thing as failure during this process. You can get right back on track if you stray from the plan and continue to feel great.

That said, I want to stress the importance of taking the commitment seriously. If you don't give the entire approach a real effort, you will not reap all the benefits. When the immune system is constantly overworking and inundated by potential relapse or flare-up triggers—such as stress, inflammatory foods, lack of exercise, lack of sleep, or environmental exposures—you may end up with poor outcomes. Think of committing wholeheartedly as improving your quality of life, while a half-hearted approach will push you toward a flare, relapse, and/or disease progression. Once you commit to lifestyle changes, you will begin to feel the benefits.

Step 2: Diet and Nutrition

It's important to choose anti-inflammatory foods that provide health-promoting nutrients your body can digest, absorb, and use while also promoting a healthy gut microbiome. The anti-inflammatory diet for MS will decrease systemic, chronic, low-grade inflammation and support a healthy immune response. Let's get started on the pantry staples that will set you up for anti-inflammatory success.

Kitchen and Pantry Clean-Out

Don't worry—you don't have to throw away everything in your cupboards. You can donate some things as you transition your pantry and kitchen to stock up for a healthy anti-inflammatory diet. Here's a general list of what should go and what can stay.

What to Cut

- Processed foods high in sodium, such as bacon, hot dogs, sausage, and snack foods
- Refined carbohydrates, such as white breads, pastries, and snacks
- Foods and desserts high in added sugar
- Deep-fried foods
- Foods high in saturated fat, such as butter, full-fat dairy, and fatty cuts of red meat
- Alcohol and caffeine

What to Keep

- Fish rich in omega-3s, such as salmon, mackerel, herring, anchovies, and sardines
- Lean protein, both plant and animal sources
- Fermented foods
- Whole grains
- Nuts, seeds, and legumes
- Mono- and polyunsaturated oils, such as olive oil, avocado oil, and sesame oil
- Herbs and spices, such as parsley, basil, oregano, cinnamon, ginger, garlic, black pepper, and turmeric

Stocking Vitamins and Supplements

When it comes to meeting your nutrient needs, my motto is food first. But some nutrients that can be beneficial when living with MS are hard to get from food alone—for example, vitamin D. Others are omega-3 DHA and EPA fatty acids. Algae-sourced DHA and EPA can be a safe supplement for those with fish allergies.

Following are some nutrients you may want to supplement. Remember: Always tell your health care provider you are considering supplements before you start. Some of them can interact with medications you may be taking or cause unusual reactions within the body.

VITAMIN D: This isn't easy to get from diet alone, which is why a supplement should be taken, especially if you live in the northern latitudes, where sun exposure is limited to a few months of the year. In addition to increasing calcium absorption and promoting bone health, vitamin D also regulates immune responses and exerts neuroprotective effects. It is best to have blood work ordered by your physician to test your serum D and adjust your dose accordingly. Ideal range for D25-OH is 50 to 100 ng/ml.

MAGNESIUM: The need for this mineral can be met from food, but additional amounts may be supplemented, as magnesium has been found to help decrease spasticity and improve sleep quality.

OMEGA-3 DHA AND EPA: Due to their anti-inflammatory qualities, these should be supplemented, especially if you're not eating fish. DHA and EPA are building blocks for immune cells called pro-resolving lipid mediators. DHA is especially important due to the neuro-protecting pro-resolving lipid mediators made from it, but both are important for immune function.

CURCUMIN: This polyphenol, which exists in turmeric, has powerful antioxidant and anti-inflammatory properties. Black pepper increases the bioavailability by 2,000 percent, according to a 2017 article published in the journal *Foods*, so make sure your supplement has both curcumin and black pepper to increase absorbability.

COQ10: An important nutrient involved in energy production, CoQ10 is also an antioxidant produced by the body, but as we age, we naturally make less. Organ meat is rich in CoQ10, which has been shown to decrease fatigue and depression in MS. If you're among the many people who don't eat organ meat regularly, a supplement may be a good idea.

FIBER: This promotes gastrointestinal health, microbiome diversity, proliferation, detoxification, and cognitive health. The by-products of our microbiome fermentation of fiber include things like energy for our enterocytes in the form of short-chain fatty acids, biotin, vitamin K, and neurotransmitters.

Preparing Your Kitchen

Stocking your kitchen with the essentials will ensure you have everything you need to make delicious anti-inflammatory meals. When you have what you need on hand, it's easier to avoid getting derailed. In the next chapter, we'll get to specific foods, but remember to vary your choices from each food group, since the synergistic effect of food is more anti-inflammatory than any one food alone. Making the healthy choice the easy choice starts with filling your kitchen with the right ingredients.

Step 3: Physical Concerns

Physical activity is an important part of adopting a lifestyle plan to manage MS. For some people, especially those used to living a very active life, physical limitations and fatigue are a primary concern.

The Importance of Movement

There is increasing evidence that physical activity and exercise can help improve MS-specific symptoms such as fatigue and depression, as well as walking, balance, cognitive function, and overall quality of life. What is even more exciting is that exercise can also have neuroprotective and neuroregenerative effects. One 2018 study published in the *Multiple Sclerosis Journal* found that engaging in progressive resistance training improved physical ability and increased brain volume. There were no additional lesions on MRI, and increased cortical thickness was found in the exercise compared to non-exercise measures.

Go at Your Own Pace

Always keep in mind your physical abilities and limitations. If you overexert yourself, it can lead to inflammation and increase fatigue. Heat intolerance is common among those with MS as well, so be sure to exercise in a cool room or when it is cooler outside. Hydration is always important, especially when exercising. If you need a reminder to drink fluids, try using a water bottle so you always know how much you've had at any point in the day.

With any exercise routine, begin slowly and gradually ease into it. Take time to warm up and cool down, and try gradually to build both duration and frequency. You might start out with just five to eight minutes and work up to 20 to 30 minutes. You may also want to start with one or two days per week and work up to three to five days. Meeting with a physical therapist who has experience with MS can be very helpful, as he or she can design an individualized plan for your unique needs and goals. Always talk with your physician before starting any exercise plans.

A number of resources are available on the National Multiple Sclerosis Society's website (nationalmssociety.org) that can help get you started with exercise, including links to exercises you can do at home. I encourage you to meet with a physical therapist or specialist who can tailor a program for you, especially if you are experiencing spasticity, lack of coordination, sensory loss, and balance problems or if you have other diagnoses that may impact your ability to exercise. Be mindful and listen to your body when engaging in physical activity or exercise of any kind. Lastly, remember to have fun!

A SIMPLE 20-MINUTE ROUTINE

Riding a recumbent bicycle is a great way to do cardio exercise safely, even if you have balance trouble, and it's easy to adjust to your preferred duration and intensity.

Warm-up: Start out with a slow pedal at very light resistance or no resistance at all. Warm up for about 5 minutes. Slowly increase the resistance to a level you can maintain for the next 8 to 10 minutes. You can increase your pedaling speed as well. Remember to listen to your body—if your muscles are telling you they are tired, decrease the resistance and cool down, even if you haven't reached the time goal.

Cooldown: Decrease your pedaling speed and resistance level, if any, to allow your heart rate and breathing to slow down to your warm-up rate before you stop pedaling. Do so by decreasing the rate at which you are pedaling, and cool down for at least 5 minutes. Once you add this exercise to your routine, you can continue to increase the time and/or resistance for a challenge.

Alternatives: If you are unable to ride a recumbent bike due to physical limitations, you can do this same routine with an arm bicycle, also known as an arm ergometer. There are also affordable mini arm-and-leg cycles that you can keep at home if you prefer to exercise there. Many can be used on the floor as a leg cycle or on the tabletop as an arm cycle. Find what works best for you and start moving.

Step 4: Mental Exercises

Physical wellness is very important, and it can even benefit your psychological health, but it is also vital to take additional steps to preserve your psychological wellness.

Psychological Wellness

Being psychologically "well" isn't the same thing as being happy and stress-free—some stress can actually be helpful. It's more about accepting yourself for who you are, building and maintaining positive relationships with others, and learning how to function effectively in your environment. Just like physical health, mental wellness requires some effort, and change does not happen overnight. Coping with physical and/or mental changes that are occurring can be difficult, especially if you don't deal with your feelings. Learning strategies to improve your mental health will help you live your best life.

Two common therapies used to improve psychological wellness are cognitive behavior therapy (CBT) and acceptance and commitment therapy (ACT). CBT is a kind of talk therapy that focuses on recognizing your thoughts and then shifting the beliefs, feelings, and even behaviors that result from those thoughts. The aim is to change the pattern of thoughts that are contributing to your emotional distress.

ACT is a type of cognitive therapy that aims to balance mindfulness and acceptance with commitment and behavior change. The goal is to reduce suffering and engage in value-guided actions. ACT and CBT are similar in that both require you to be aware of your feelings and ultimately shift your thoughts. A 2018 study published in the *International Journal of Body, Mind, and Culture* found both of these treatment options to be effective therapies for reducing depression in women with MS.

Mindfulness, Meditation, and Stress Reduction

An additional activity that may improve your mental well-being is mindfulness, which may be a buzzword now but is more than just a fad. Both CBT and ACT require mindfulness, which simply means actively paying attention to the present moment—including your current thoughts, physical sensations, and surroundings—and not allowing yourself to become overly reactive. One way to practice mindfulness is through meditation. A 2014 systematic review of so-called mindfulness-based interventions in MS, published in the journal *BMC Neurology*, found them to be a benefit to quality of life, mental health, and some physical health measures.

Psychological stress can affect you physically, leading to increased inflammation, and may even exacerbate MS symptoms such as fatigue. Being mindful of your feelings and stress levels is an important part of managing your stress.

Dealing with Feelings

When someone I am working with shares strong feelings with me, I ask them to imagine I am someone they are close with. This lets them reflect on how that person might feel after hearing those original feelings. Just having someone listen to you can help you start to feel better, and ideally you have a close relative or friend with whom you can share such feelings.

Support groups can also be useful. Try to find a local MS Society group or other local nonprofit group. If they don't exist in your area, you can always join an online group. Getting to know new people and hearing their stories can be inspiring. You can learn a lot from others, and at the same time, they can learn from you. Helping others can improve your psychological wellness, too—you may join a group looking for support and soon find you're part of a support network for others.

A SIMPLE MEDITATION

This simple meditation can be used to help you relax, fall asleep, or reduce stress.

Start in a comfortable seated position or lie down on the floor. Next, close your eyes and continue to breathe naturally. Pay attention to your breathing without trying to control it. Begin to notice how your body moves as you inhale and exhale. Become aware of the movement in your belly, chest, and shoulders. You may rest your hands on your belly or chest or just comfortably by your sides. Your mind will likely wander—when it does, just bring your focus back to your breath.

Practice this for 2 to 3 minutes at a time at first. Increase the duration as you become more comfortable with the process. You may want to start with a guided meditation using your smartphone or computer. Alternatively, you might find meditation books at the library for tips that can help you master your practice. There may even be a local meditation instructor in your area who can teach you diaphragmatic breathing, comfortable postures, and relaxation and concentration techniques.

Step 5: Prepare for the Journey

You are about to embark on a big life change—it's perfectly normal to feel a mix of excitement and apprehension. Just remember to focus on each step without projecting future obstacles that may never arise.

Routines Help

We are all creatures of habit, and whenever you commit to a behavior change, it means a change in your routine. Depending on your current lifestyle, implementing this anti-inflammatory approach may seem like a difficult feat. You have been working on your habits your whole life, and now you may have to change some, or many, of them. Having a routine will make it easier to stick to the behavior changes recommended in this anti-inflammatory diet approach. It is very important to persist with the changes so that you can feel the benefits and start improving your health. Having a few healthy foods once in a while will not significantly improve your health, but having a healthy diet pattern and lifestyle will.

Carve Out Time

While I have made the diet as easy as possible, you will still need to dedicate some time to implementing the program. I recommend choosing one or two days of the week when you have extra time for meal planning and prepping. For example, if you know you have free time on Tuesdays, batch cook a meal or two to save you time and energy on other days. Alternatively, you can commit to doing as much as possible when your energy levels are high. This is your journey, and part of the journey is figuring out the best route for you.

Stumbles and Backslides

You will likely experience some stumbles along the way. Don't worry; this is expected. It doesn't mean that the entire journey has been derailed—it simply means you need to change course and get back on track. Don't feel bad or guilty about a slipup. Sometimes you may just need a cue to help trigger your new behavior. For example, if you are having trouble keeping adequately hydrated, you could leave your water pitcher out on the counter to serve as a reminder to have a glass of water every time you see it.

If you stray from the diet, just commit to getting back on track. Maybe your meditation practice has stopped for a few weeks. Try leaving yourself a sticky-note reminder to meditate in the room where you would normally meditate until it becomes habit again. Be patient with the process and yourself. Remember that behavior change is not easy, but nothing worthwhile ever is.

Let Yourself Enjoy It

While behavior change isn't easy, it can be fun. Trying new foods and recipes can be an adventure. Being creative and experimenting with different combinations of flavors can yield some pretty delicious results. I encourage you to experiment with recipes, make modifications based on your preferences, and share your creations with others. You can share them online via social media or at your table with friends and good conversation.

Try different techniques for your meditation practice. Maybe try it sitting up one day and lying down another. You can find guided meditations that you can do anywhere online or on a smartphone app. Let yourself enjoy the journey.

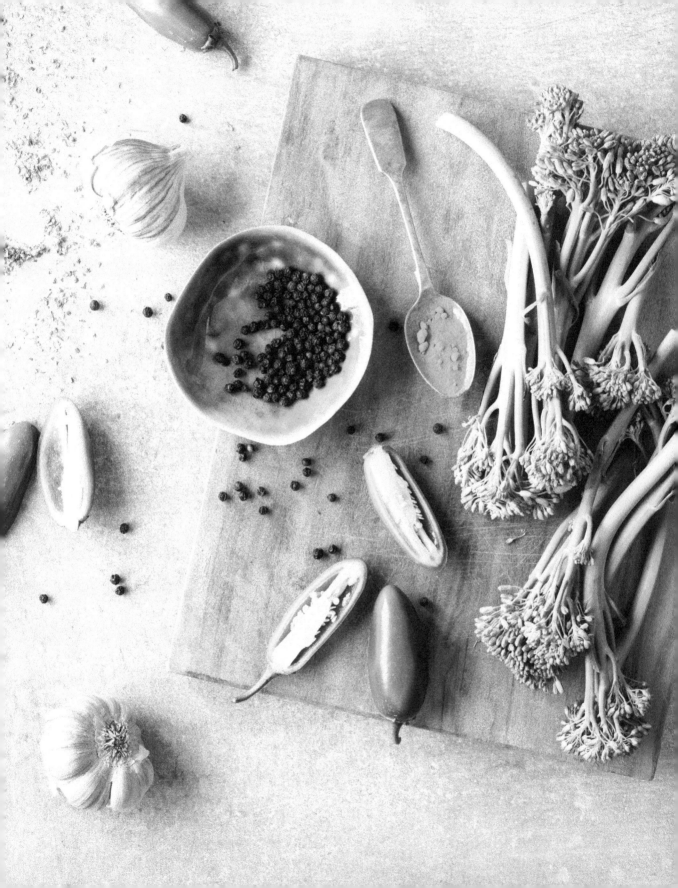

CHAPTER THREE

The Meal Plan

In this chapter, you will find 28 days of meal suggestions for breakfast, lunch, and dinner to help you stick to an anti-inflammatory diet. This meal plan is designed to be mindful of your everyday schedule and physical limitations. There are easy recipes and plenty of meal-prep suggestions, making grab-and-go a healthy option.

You don't have to spend hours in the kitchen to adopt an anti-inflammatory diet. Many of the meals can be prepared in 30 minutes or less. The slow-cooker meals allow you to spend minimal time in active meal preparation. You can use these recipes when you know you have limited time, but remember that doing so takes a little planning. You may need to start your slow cooker in the morning before work. Looking ahead at the meal plan and moving meals around to fit your lifestyle will allow you flexibility and make it easier to follow the plan.

Restocking

Remember the pantry clean-out from the previous chapter? Now it's time to restock the refrigerator and pantry with MS-friendly foods. Let's start with the basic staples you will want on hand. Please choose organic or wild when possible. See the Dirty Dozen and the Clean Fifteen™ (page 195) to help you decide which produce should be organic.

Restocking pantry staples may take some time. I would start here and move on to the four-week plan once you feel you have all the new pantry staples. Having the ingredients in the following list on hand will keep your grocery shopping to just fresh produce and proteins.

Pantry Staples: These amounts will vary depending on your household size. The pantry staples include all food groups so that you can throw together a tasty, well-balanced meal even if you can't get to the store for fresh protein or produce. The amounts listed are my initial quantity recommendations. After the four-week plan, you can shift amounts based on your preferences.

- **Oils:** 16 ounces extra-virgin olive oil, 16 ounces avocado oil, 5 ounces toasted sesame oil (amount you would use in 3 to 4 months)

- **Nut/Seed Butter:** 16 ounces of natural peanut butter, almond butter, sunflower seed butter

- **Nuts/Seeds:** 2 cups each of almonds, walnuts, and cashews; 1 pound ground flaxseed; 1 pound ground chia; 1 cup sesame seeds; 1 cup pumpkin seeds

- **Spices/Dried Herbs:** turmeric, black pepper, Himalayan salt, oregano, basil, cumin, cayenne or chili powder, onion powder, garlic powder, sage, tarragon, curry powder, dill, dried lemon peel

- **Sauces:** (these can all be found gluten-free) small jar mayonnaise made with olive oil, low-sodium soy sauce, low-sodium broth, low-sugar barbecue sauce, Szechuan sauce; Optional: minced garlic

- **Whole Grains:** 16 ounces brown rice, 16 ounces quinoa, 2 pounds old-fashioned rolled oats, 14½ ounces whole-grain or legume pasta

- **Canned/Packaged:** 3 cans each of black beans, white beans, kidney beans; 1 (3-ounce) pouch smoked salmon; 1 (15-ounce) can chicken; 1 (10-pack) nori; 5 to 6 ounces miso (white or red)
- **Dried:** 6 ounces of dried fruits, such as cherries

- **Sweeteners/Baking:** real maple syrup, raw honey, coconut sugar, cinnamon, vanilla extract, other extracts you prefer, baking powder, baking soda
- **Frozen:** 16 ounces broccoli, cauliflower, snow peas, carrots, onion and pepper blend, and your choice of mixed vegetables; 12 ounces mixed berries; 12 ounces frozen fish (2 servings)

Fruits and Veggies

You don't have to purchase every vegetable—the key is to have variety, so I've offered plenty of choices. You will want to choose from each of the three categories, aiming for 2 or more servings from each daily. Shopping seasonally will help you rotate among the following options.

Serving size: ½ cup, or 1 cup for raw leafy greens

LEAFY GREENS	CRUCIFEROUS/ SULFUR-RICH	COLORFUL
Arugula	Broccoli	Avocado
Beet greens	Brussels sprouts	Bell peppers
Chard	Cabbage	Beets
Collard greens	Cauliflower	Blueberries
Dandelion greens	Garlic	Carrots
Kale	Kale	Celery
Romaine	Onions	Cucumber
Spinach	Turnips	Green beans
Watercress		Oranges
		Radish
		Raspberries
		Squash
		Strawberries
		Sweet potato

Proteins

Plant-based proteins, which provide fiber and phytonutrients, should also be part of your diet pattern. There are plenty of varieties of omega-3-rich fish to allow you to choose whatever is on sale. Animal proteins should be lean and low-sodium without preservatives.

PLANT PROTEIN (~ ½ cup)	**OMEGA-3-RICH FISH** (4 to 5 ounces)	**ANIMAL MEAT** (3 to 4 ounces)
Frozen shelled edamame	Halibut	Chicken (skinless)
Nuts/seeds/ legumes (¼ to ½ cup)	Herring	Lamb
Organic tempeh	Mackerel	Lean beef
Organic tofu	Salmon	Lean pork
Spirulina (optional)	Sardines, anchovies	Sausage (low-sodium, no additives)
	Sea bass	Turkey
	Tuna	

Dairy/Dairy Alternatives

Dairy is an important source of calcium and vitamin D. Try to purchase dairy alternatives that are fortified with calcium and vitamin D (unsweetened is preferred).

DAIRY	**MILK ALTERNATIVES**	**YOGURT**
Kefir	Almond, coconut, flaxseed, hazelnut, hemp, oat, and soy	Cultured milk, coconut milk, almond milk, and soy milk
Low-fat milk		

FOODS TO ADORE, FOODS TO AVOID

By this point, you have a pretty good understanding that the foods we eat can impact our wellness, influence our immune response, and be anti-inflammatory or inflammatory. Here's a quick reference of foods you want to eat often and foods that can be harmful to your health.

FOODS TO ADORE

Avocados
Cruciferous vegetables
Dark, leafy greens
Deeply colored fruits and vegetables
  (berries, carrots, etc.)
Fermented foods
  (yogurt, kefir, kombucha, kimchi)
Legumes
Mushrooms
Nuts
Olive oil
Omega-3-rich fish
Seeds
Whole grains

FOODS TO AVOID

Any fully or partially hydrogenated oil
Any intolerances/allergens
  (e.g., dairy, gluten)
Corn oil
Deep-fried foods
Excess alcohol
Excess caffeine
High-sodium foods (>20 percent DV on
  the label)
Refined grains, refined baked goods
Refined safflower oil
Refined sugar
Regular peanut butter (it has hydroge-
  nated oil)

Things You'll Need

You can make things easy by keeping all the equipment you need on hand.

Pots and Pans

- 8-by-8-inch and/or 9-by-13-inch baking dish—great for any use, especially when you need a larger rim (frittata, casserole, brownies)
- 11-by-17-inch rimmed baking sheet—great for both cookies and vegetables
- Blender or food processor
- Large soup pan or stockpot with a lid
- Medium and large skillets for sautéing vegetables and proteins
- Medium saucepan with a lid for heating soups and sauces
- Roasting pan—useful for roasting whole chicken, turkey, beef
- Silicone lids for pots and pans of any size
- Slow cooker, which cuts down on active cooking time and makes batch cooking easier

Utensils

- Cutting boards—always place a towel underneath when using to prevent sliding
- Glass or stainless-steel mixing bowls—could also be used for storage
- Measuring cups for both solids and liquids
- Measuring spoons
- Meat thermometer
- Metal or wooden skewers
- Sharp knives—they are safer because a dull knife increases the chance of slipping and cutting yourself
- Silicone ladle
- Silicone serving spoons
- Silicone spatula
- Slotted serving spoon
- Tongs

Storage Solutions

- Baking dishes and glass or silicone storage containers in various sizes with lids
- Beeswax wraps
- Burlap sacks for root vegetables
- Freezer bags
- Mason jars
- Mixing bowls with lids
- Reusable snack and sandwich bags
- Reusable storage containers in various sizes

SHOPPING TIPS

Grocery shopping can be stressful when you're in a hurry or are looking for new ingredients—especially if you're also feeling fatigue, having a flare-up, or managing a physical limitation. To make things easier, try to plan when you shop so that it doesn't become a hurried, last-minute trip. Give yourself time to calmly navigate the store and find everything.

Organizing your shopping list based on the layout of the store is very helpful as well. Maybe you start with fresh produce, go on to inner-aisle items such as canned goods, and then get fresh protein and frozen foods. It will depend on your store's layout, but I've tried to keep the shopping lists organized to reduce the time you spend going back and forth in the store.

Alternatively, you may find shopping online is easier. You can have the order ready to pick up on your way home or possibly have it delivered. Try to dress appropriately as well—most stores are cold, and if you are uncomfortable while shopping, it may cause you to rush and forget some items.

Week One

This anti-inflammatory meal plan starts out with less complicated recipes. Most of this week's recipes don't require any cooking and include leftovers to keep prep and shopping time to a minimum. Leftovers will be marked "LO."

The first week introduces more anti-inflammatory foods than you may be used to eating, but the ingredients are all easy to find. If you haven't started restocking your pantry, you may want to add some of the optional pantry staples as well. If there is anything you do not want to try, substitute another recipe from the book.

Coffee is okay, but limit your intake and drink plenty of hydrating fluids. Your exact fluid needs will vary depending on your age, size, and other health conditions. We need fluids to help with digestion and absorption of nutrients, transport of nutrients to cells, regulation of body temperature, maintenance of blood volume, excretion of bacteria and other toxins, and prevention of constipation.

Hydration is important even during winter months when we are not sweating as much. Even mild dehydration can affect cognitive function and lead to muscle weakness, increased fatigue, and other symptoms. If you are experiencing bladder dysfunction, it is important that you do not restrict fluids. Doing so can lead to increased fatigue, as well as increased risk of urinary tract infections. Please increase fluid intake slowly to get your body used to extra fluids.

Note: The Make-Ahead Farmers'-Market-Finds Frittata (page 69) makes 8 servings. Keep 3 servings for this week and store the remaining frittata in the freezer. Cut into individual squares, wrap in wax paper, freeze completely, and then wrap the squares in foil and place them inside a freezer bag. You will reheat them individually in the microwave in the coming weeks.

Shopping List

PRODUCE:

Apples (3)

Avocados (3)

Basil (1 bunch)

Beet (1)

Bell peppers, mixed colors (3)

Cabbage, red (1 head)

Carrots, shredded and bagged
 (10 ounces)

Celery (1 bunch)

Cucumbers (3)

Curly kale (1 bunch)

Fennel (1 bulb)

Mushrooms (6 ounces)

Onions, red (2)

Onion, yellow (1)

Parsley (1 bunch)

Spinach, bagged (1 pound)

Sweet potato (1)

Tomatoes (4 medium)

Tomatoes, cherry (1 pint)

DAIRY (OPTIONAL):

Feta cheese (6 ounces)

Kefir, plain (1 quart)

Mexican-blend cheese, shredded
 (8 ounces)

Mozzarella, fresh (4 ounces)

Mozzarella, shredded (8 ounces)

MEAT, POULTRY, FISH, AND EGGS:

Chicken, 2 (12½-ounce) cans

Chicken sausage, low-sodium, low-fat
 (1 package)

Eggs (1 dozen)

Smoked salmon, 1 (3-ounce) pouch

FROZEN:

Artichoke hearts, 1 (12-ounce) bag

Asparagus, 1 (12-ounce) bag

Blueberries, 1 (12-ounce) bag

Strawberries, 1 (12-ounce) bag

OTHER:

Almond milk, unsweetened vanilla
 (1 gallon)

Coconut flakes, unsweetened
 (4 ounces)

Flatbread wraps, Flatout brand (1 bag)

Hummus, 1 (10-ounce) container

Peanut butter, natural, 1 (16-ounce) jar

	BREAKFAST	LUNCH	
MONDAY	PB&J Smoothie (page 67)	Avocado-Chicken Pinwheels (page 155)	
TUESDAY	Berry-licious Overnight Oats (page 71)	LO Easy Chicken Sausage and Cucumber Salad (page 156)	
WEDNESDAY	Easy Breakfast Hash (page 75)	LO Avocado-Chicken Pinwheels (page 155)	
THURSDAY	Make-Ahead Farmers'-Market-Finds Frittata (page 69)	LO Make-Ahead Sesame-Soy Edamame Bowl (page 114)	
FRIDAY	PB&J Smoothie (page 67)	Smoked Salmon Grain Bowl (page 147)	
SATURDAY	LO Make-Ahead Farmers'-Market-Finds Frittata (page 69)	Rainbow Pinwheels (page 130)	
SUNDAY	LO Make-Ahead Farmers'-Market-Finds Frittata (page 69)	Grain Salad with Dried Plums (page 111)	

SNACK	DINNER	ACTIVITY SUGGESTIONS
1 apple and ¼ cup almonds	Easy Chicken Sausage and Cucumber Salad (page 156)	1 minute mindfulness routine
2 celery stalks with ¼ cup hummus	Baked Lemon Halibut with Artichokes (page 137)	5 minutes stretching and/or physical activity
½ cup raspberries and ¼ cup almonds	Make-Ahead Sesame-Soy Edamame Bowl (page 114)	2 minutes mindfulness routine
1 apple and 1 tablespoon peanut butter	LO Easy Chicken Sausage and Cucumber Salad (page 156)	6 minutes stretching or physical activity
2 to 3 celery stalks and ¼ cup hummus	Easy Caprese Pasta Salad (page 121)	3 minutes mindfulness routine
½ cup raspberries and ¼ cup almonds	LO Baked Lemon Halibut with Artichokes (page 137)	8 minutes stretching or physical activity
1 apple and 1 tablespoon peanut butter	LO Easy Caprese Pasta Salad (page 121)	3 minutes mindfulness routine

Weekly Check-In

Find your written or audio journal and add to it now. After one week of lifestyle changes, how are you feeling? How have you done with the mindfulness activities? Have you tried to redirect any negative thinking, and if so, how did it work for you?

How are you doing with meal preparation, and are you enjoying the meals? Record any changes you may have experienced, such as gastrointestinal symptoms (bowel habits, gas, bloating, etc.) and fatigue severity. Have you experienced any barriers to successfully implementing this plan? If so, how do you think you can modify the plan to succeed? Aim to clear any obstacles so that you can make this plan work for you. Consider talking with a friend, family member, or health care provider about the barriers, as they may be able to help.

Week Two

Week two will add more anti-inflammatory foods to your meal plan. Again, this may mean a few more vegetables than you are used to, but stick with it. They are loaded with anti-inflammatory phytonutrients, vitamins, minerals, and fiber. I have tried to keep shopping lists to a minimum, so leftovers are included here as well. If you are making a recipe that creates larger quantities, freeze the leftovers to start stocking your freezer with ready-to-go meals. This can set you up for success even after the four-week plan ends.

Keep in mind the activity suggestions are just suggestions. You can look back at your journal entries and decide what exercise to do and for how long. If the routines were difficult, consider decreasing the suggested time and work toward increasing the time next week. Set your own personal goals and write them in your journal. Drink plenty of hydrating fluids daily, and aim for 8 ounces of almond milk each day.

Shopping List

PRODUCE:

Apple (1)

Avocado (1)

Bell peppers, red (2)

Celery (1 bunch)

Cilantro (1 bunch)

Cucumber (1)

Garlic (1 head)

Lemon (1)

Lentils, presteamed (8 ounces)

Mushrooms (8 ounces)

Mushrooms, portobello (2)

Onion, red (1)

Onion, yellow (1)

Oranges (2)

Potato, purple (1)

Sage (1 bunch)

Sweet potato (1)

Tomatoes, cherry (1 pint)

Watermelon (about 5 pounds)

Zucchini (1)

DAIRY (OPTIONAL):

Feta cheese (if you purchased it last week, you will have enough left)

Goat cheese (4 ounces)

MEAT, POULTRY, FISH, AND EGGS:

Chicken, 1 (12½-ounce) can

Chicken breast, 1 large (about 9½ ounces)

Eggs (6)

Smoked salmon, 1 (3-ounce) pouch

Tempeh, 1 package

FROZEN:

Corn, 1 (10-ounce) bag

Green beans, 1 (16-ounce) bag

Onion-and-bell-pepper blend, 1 (14- to 16-ounce) bag

Snow peas, 1 (10-ounce) bag

OTHER:

Almond milk, unsweetened (½ gallon)

Bread, whole-grain (1 loaf)

Coconut milk, light (1 can)

Corn tortillas (6)

Pumpkin purée (1 can)

Refried beans, vegetarian, 1 (15-ounce) can

Sesame-ginger dressing, 1 (12-ounce) bottle

Tomato soup, low-sodium (1 carton)

	BREAKFAST	LUNCH	
MONDAY	LO Make-Ahead Farmers'-Market-Finds Frittata (page 69)	Comforting Grilled Cheese and Tomato Soup (page 120)	
TUESDAY	Spiced Pumpkin Oatmeal (page 72)	LO Waldorf Chicken Salad Sandwich (page 154)	
WEDNESDAY	Berry Refresh Smoothie (page 66)	Roasted Veggie Tacos (page 124)	
THURSDAY	Spiced Pumpkin Oatmeal (page 72)	Black Bean Taco Salad (page 115)	
FRIDAY	Savory Quinoa Breakfast Bowl (page 76)	Thai Tempeh Lettuce Wraps (page 125)	
SATURDAY	Salmon-Avocado Toast (page 73)	LO Thai Tempeh Lettuce Wraps (page 125)	
SUNDAY	Savory Quinoa Breakfast Bowl (page 76)	LO Savory Lentil-Bruschetta Shrooms (page 123)	

SNACK	DINNER	ACTIVITY SUGGESTIONS
½ cup Crisp Roasted Chickpeas (page 82)	Waldorf Chicken Salad Sandwich (page 154)	3 minutes mindfulness routine
1 orange and ¼ cup walnuts	LO Comforting Grilled Cheese and Tomato Soup (page 120)	8 minutes stretching or physical activity
LO ½ cup Crisp Roasted Chickpeas (page 82)	Lemon-Turmeric Chicken Breast (page 157)	4 minutes mindfulness routine
Cooling Mint-Watermelon Salad (page 107)	LO Roasted Veggie Tacos (page 124) and LO Lemon-Turmeric Chicken Breast (page 157)	8 minutes stretching or physical activity
LO Cooling Mint-Watermelon Salad (page 107)	LO Black Bean Taco Salad (page 115)	5 minutes mindfulness routine
1 orange and ¼ cup walnuts	Savory Lentil-Bruschetta Shrooms (page 123)	10 minutes stretching or physical activity
LO Cooling Mint-Watermelon Salad (page 107)	Baked Lemon Halibut with Artichokes (page 137)	5 minutes mindfulness routine

Weekly Check-In

Take some time to reflect. Maybe you are getting into a routine and forming new habits around meal times and food prepping. Check in with how you feel about the changes you have made to your diet and lifestyle. Are there parts that you really enjoy? Are you having difficulty with anything? Are you seeing any improvements in bowel habits or changes in energy level? Did you remember to hydrate?

Are you feeling good about the hard work you have put in this far? You should be! Take a minute to recognize the work you are putting in to improve your health and feel better. Remember that you deserve recognition for all that you are doing.

Week Three

You're a whole two weeks into your commitment. This week, you may start to see even more new ingredients. If you have never cooked with tofu before, the dill dip is a delicious recipe to start with—it's one of my absolute favorite things to dip veggies in. There are also some sweet treats this week, with black beans to provide some fiber and help control blood sugar.

Shopping List

PRODUCE:

Arugula, 1 (5-ounce) bag
Bell peppers, red and yellow (1 each)
Cabbage, purple, shredded (8 ounces)
Carrots, baby, 1 (12-ounce) bag
Carrots, shredded (10 ounces)
Cucumber (1)
Dill weed, fresh (1 bunch)
Ginger, fresh, 1 (2-inch) piece
Kale (12 ounces)
Lemon (1)

Mushrooms (5 ounces)
Onion, yellow (1)
Orange (1)
Potato, red (1)
Scallions (4 ounces)
Spinach, 1 (6-ounce) bag
Strawberries (16 ounces)
Sweet potato (1)
Zucchini (2)

DAIRY (OPTIONAL):

Parmesan cheese (½ cup)

Yogurt, plain low-fat (32 ounces)

MEAT, POULTRY, FISH, AND EGGS:

Anchovies, 1 (2-ounce) can
Eggs (6)
Shrimp, medium deveined (1 pound)
Smoked salmon, 1 (3-ounce) pouch

Halibut, frozen (12 ounces)
Tempeh (1 package)
Tofu, silken (14 ounces)
Tuna (8 ounces)

FROZEN:

Avocado chunks (10 ounces)
Berries, mixed (16 ounces)
Broccoli and cauliflower florets
  (16 ounces)

Edamame, shelled (12 ounces)
Peaches (16 ounces)

OTHER:

Almond milk, unsweetened (½ gallon)
Black beans, 1 (15-ounce) can
Cocoa powder, raw (8 ounces)

Mustard, Dijon (12 ounces)
Worcestershire sauce (5 ounces)
Sesame seeds (2 tablespoons)

	BREAKFAST	LUNCH	
MONDAY	Creamy Chocolate-Berry Smoothie (page 68)	Classic Caesar Salad (page 109)	
TUESDAY	Cinnamon-Peach Overnight Oats (page 70)	Bomb Diggity Dill Salmon Salad (page 112)	
WEDNESDAY	Creamy Chocolate-Berry Smoothie (page 68)	Strawberry-Spinach Salad (page 106)	
THURSDAY	LO Cinnamon-Peach Overnight Oats (page 70)	Make-Ahead Sesame-Soy Edamame Bowl (page 114) and rice	
FRIDAY	LO Make-Ahead Farmers'-Market-Finds Frittata (page 69)	LO Sesame-Ginger Halibut and Mushrooms (page 138)	
SATURDAY	LO Make-Ahead Farmers'-Market-Finds Frittata (page 69)	LO Savory Sage Tuna with Baked Potato and Vegetables (page 142)	
SUNDAY	PB&J Smoothie (page 67)	LO Warm Kale Salad (page 113)	

SNACK	DINNER	ACTIVITY SUGGESTIONS
Bomb Diggity Dill Dip (page 83) and 1 cup celery and carrots	LO Classic Caesar Salad (page 109) and 4 to 6 medium shrimp	1 minute mindfulness routine
½ cup strawberries and ¼ cup almonds	Sesame-Ginger Halibut and Mushrooms (page 138)	5 minutes stretching and/or physical activity
LO Bomb Diggity Dill Dip (page 83) and 1 cup sliced bell peppers	Creole Shrimp Kebabs (page 150)	2 minutes mindfulness routine
Black Bean Brownie (page 175) and 2 strawberries	LO Creole Shrimp Kebabs (page 150)	6 minutes stretching or physical activity
1 orange and ¼ cup walnuts	Savory Sage Tuna with Baked Potato and Vegetables (page 142)	3 minutes mindfulness routine
LO Black Bean Brownie (page 175) and 1 glass soy or almond milk	Warm Kale Salad (page 113)	8 minutes stretching or physical activity
Black Bean Brownie (page 175) and 1 glass soy or almond milk	Barbecue Tempeh Bowl (page 128)	3 minutes mindfulness routine

Weekly Check-In

Remember to check in weekly. Use your journal or cell phone to record how you feel week three went. If there were any favorite recipes, jot them down for future use. Also, remember you can check the recipes section for more options, especially if you have been craving something specific. For example, there's a ceviche recipe I love in the seafood chapter, but I didn't include it in the four-week plan.

Week Four

This is your final week, but you can reuse the plan as much as you would like or swap in additional recipes for more variety. You should be getting more comfortable in the kitchen and have some kind of routine in place by now. Getting your groceries is probably becoming a regular habit. Most of the weeks have used a lot of the usual suspects, such as green leafy vegetables, onions, garlic, and peppers. While there are many anti-inflammatory foods, you have already had most of these, so you should be feeling more comfortable preparing them.

Shopping List

PRODUCE:

Apple (1)

Arugula, 1 (5-ounce) bag

Avocados (2)

Bananas (2)

Beets (4)

Beets, roasted, 1 (8-ounce) package

Broccoli (1 head)

Cauliflower (1 head)

Cherries, dried tart (3 ounces)

Cilantro, fresh (1 bunch)

Clementines (4)

Curly kale (6 ounces)

Fennel (1 bulb)

Garlic (1 bulb)

Lime (1)

Mixed greens, 1 (16-ounce) bag

Mushrooms (14 ounces)

Onions, white (2)

Onion, yellow (1)

Oranges (4)

Parsley, fresh (1 bunch)

Radishes (2)

Rosemary, fresh (1 bunch)
Spinach, 2 (16-ounce) bags
Sweet potatoes (2 pounds)

Tomatoes, cherry (1 pint)
Tomatoes, sun-dried, 1 (3-ounce) bag
Zucchini (2 large)

DAIRY (OPTIONAL):

Goat cheese (4 ounces)

Yogurt, nonfat plain Greek (32 ounces)

MEAT, POULTRY, FISH, AND EGGS:

Beef, lean ground (16 ounces)
Pork shoulder, boneless (4 pounds)
Salmon (12 ounces)

Salmon, smoked, 1 (3-ounce) pouch
Turkey, lean ground (3 pounds)

FROZEN:

Broccoli florets, 1 (12-ounce) bag
Cauliflower florets, 1 (12-ounce) bag
Cauliflower rice, 1 (12-ounce) bag
Mango chunks, 1 (16-ounce) bag

Onion-and-bell-pepper blend,
  1 (14- to 16-ounce) bag
Pineapple chunks, 1 (16-ounce) bag

OTHER:

Almond milk, unsweetened (½ gallon)
Black beans, 1 (15-ounce) can
Bread, whole-grain (½ loaf)
Cannellini beans, 4 (15½-ounce) cans
Chicken broth, low-sodium,
  1 (32-ounce) carton
Chickpeas, 1 (15½-ounce) can
Chiles, diced green, 1 (4.4-ounce) can
Coconut extract
Cumin seeds
Farro, 1 (18-ounce) package

Garam masala
Hemp seeds
Pasta, gluten-free, 1 (1-pound) box
Pesto, 1 (6- or 8-ounce) jar
Pumpkin seeds
Salsa (1 jar)
Spaghetti, whole-grain, 1 (1-pound) box
Tofu, extra-firm (16 ounces)
Tomato purée, 1 (15½-ounce) can
Tortillas, corn, 1 (8-count) package

	BREAKFAST	LUNCH	
MONDAY	Green Goodness Smoothie (page 64)	LO Barbecue Tempeh Bowl (page 128)	
TUESDAY	LO Salmon-Avocado Toast (page 73)	Simple Miso Soup (page 100)	
WEDNESDAY	Green Goodness Smoothie (page 64)	Superfood Salad (page 108)	
THURSDAY	Southwest Tofu Scramble (page 74)	LO 50/50 Mushroom Burger (page 166) and Baked Sweet Potato Wedges (page 88)	
FRIDAY	Piña Kale-ada Smoothie (page 65)	LO Broccoli Macaroni "Alfredo" (page 118)	
SATURDAY	LO Southwest Tofu Scramble (page 74)	LO Slow-Cooker Turkey and White Bean Chili (page 159)	
SUNDAY	Piña Kale-ada Smoothie (page 65)	LO Chana Masala over Cauliflower "Rice" (page 129)	

SNACK	DINNER	ACTIVITY SUGGESTIONS
Beet and Goat Cheese Tartines (page 84)	Almond-Pesto-Crusted Salmon (page 146)	1 minute mindfulness routine
LO Beet and Goat Cheese Tartines (page 84)	Smoked Salmon Grain Bowl (page 147)	5 minutes stretching and/or physical activity
½ avocado, sliced, with freshly ground black pepper and turmeric	50/50 Mushroom Burger (page 166) and Baked Sweet Potato Wedges (page 88)	2 minutes mindfulness routine
1 orange and ¼ cup pumpkin seeds	Broccoli Macaroni "Alfredo" (page 118) and LO Superfood Salad (page 108)	6 minutes stretching and/or physical activity
2 Chocolate-Coconut Truffles (page 177)	Slow-Cooker Turkey and White Bean Chili (page 159)	3 minutes mindfulness routine
1 orange and ¼ cup pumpkin seeds	Chana Masala over Cauliflower "Rice" (page 129)	8 minutes stretching and/or physical activity
2 LO Chocolate-Coconut Truffles (page 177)	Slow-Cooker Carnitas (page 164)	3 minutes mindfulness routine

Weekly Check-In

Take time to reflect after week four. Think about whether you would like to continue on this plan or use the recipes section to start making new weekly meal plans. Keep the recipes varied and try to choose meals that may have some similar ingredients to keep your shopping list as short as possible. Maybe you can even start switching some proteins around and make your own new recipes.

Making Adjustments

As MS can lead to many physical limitations in addition to fatigue, I have tried to keep the prep time down. I also wanted to include fresh produce for those who want to purchase seasonal fruits and vegetables. I've made recommendations on many of the recipes to make them easier. For example, using frozen chopped vegetables makes most of the recipes very easy to prep. Minced ginger and garlic are both options, and even buying shredded carrots and cabbage helps.

Feel free to modify any of the recipes further if you have limitations that prevent you from using certain ingredients or tools in the kitchen. When buying foods that have been precut, just make sure that they do not have sauces or spices added. Many times, the added flavors also add sodium and sugar, which can increase inflammation.

Regulating your temperature is another consideration. Keeping a glass of ice water nearby or adjusting the thermostat before cooking can help manage sensitivity to heat. A cooling towel is a great help as well. Keep a chair close by in the kitchen so you can take a quick break if you feel fatigued after you've started cooking. It's better to take a rest instead of overexerting yourself.

You may also find it helpful to reorganize your pantry staples to keep close the items you use the most. For those who are cooking from a wheelchair and are unable to see into the pot or pan, a mounted mirror might be helpful. If any of your physical limitations are new, I recommend having an occupational therapist come to your home to assess your environment. He or she may suggest helpful tools like adaptive cutting boards or utensils.

About the Recipes

These recipes are for healthy, anti-inflammatory foods that don't skimp on flavor. Many of them will only take 30 minutes to prepare, and the slow-cooker recipes allow you to do other things while the cooker does the work. Some may stretch your palate a little and include ingredients you may not typically use. There may be new proteins, vegetables, or spices in this diet pattern—just be adventurous and enjoy the experience!

While some of the ingredients may be new or something you have not cooked with in years, they won't be difficult to find and they won't be expensive. Check the bulk section at your local grocery store—it's a great way to save money and allows you to purchase just the amount you need. Some of my favorites to buy in bulk include nuts, seeds, spices, dried herbs, legumes, and whole grains.

After four weeks on the plan, you now have an idea of what a balanced, anti-inflammatory diet looks like. You can add your own style and preferences and modify some of the recipes. I once heard the famous chef Jacques Pépin say to always make a recipe first according to how it's written. Then, once you have made it, you can alter it to make it your own. This, of course, does not apply if you have an allergy or intolerance and need to avoid a specific food.

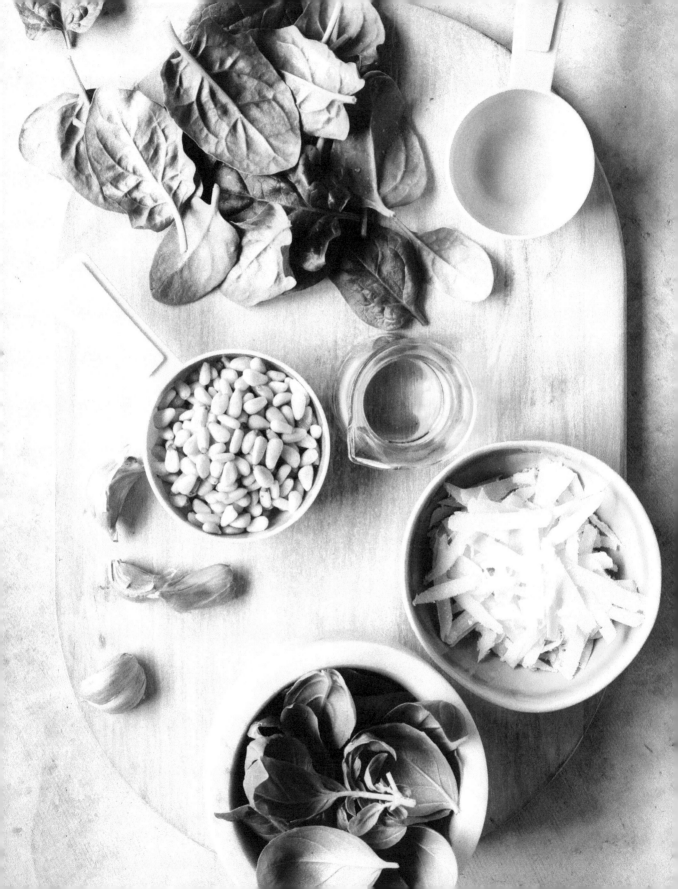

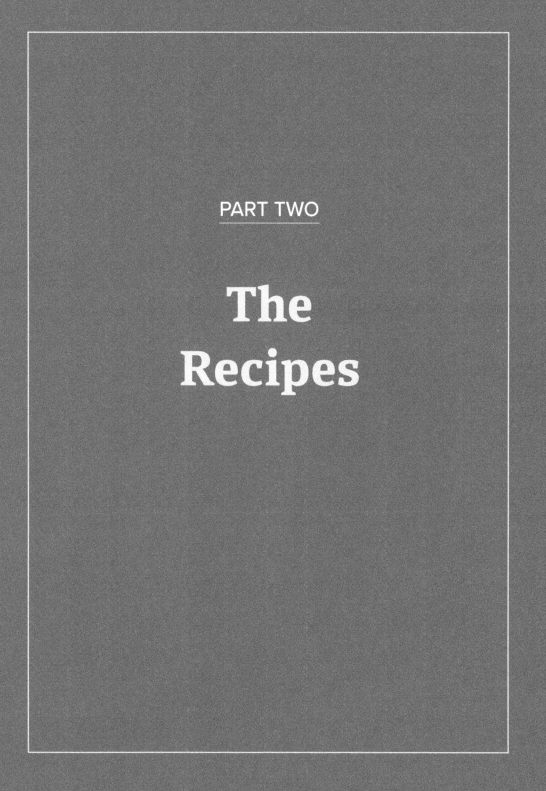

PART TWO

The Recipes

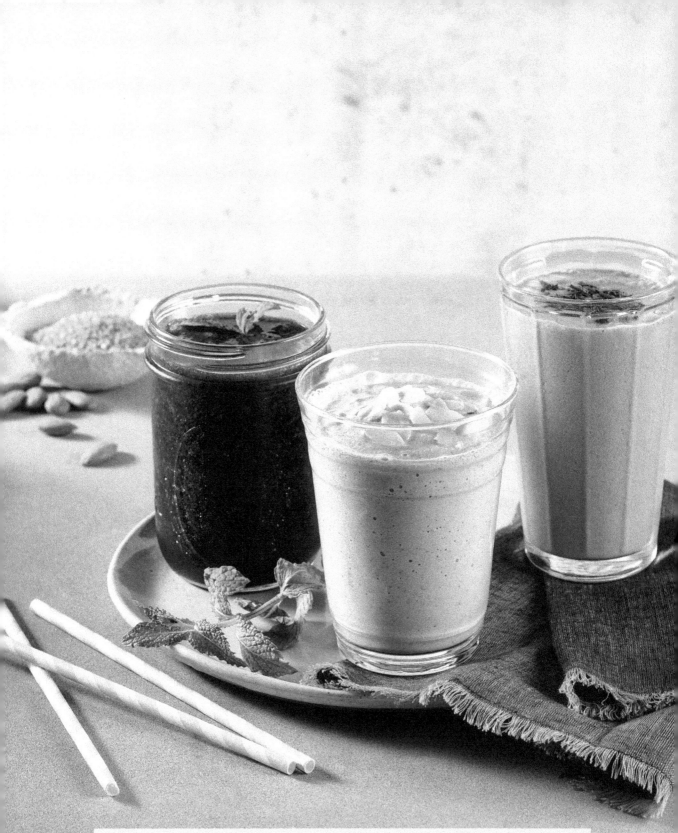

Berry Refresh Smoothie Page 66 | Green Goodness Smoothie Page 64 | Creamy Chocolate-Berry Smoothie Page 68

CHAPTER FOUR

Breakfast and Smoothies

Berry Smoothie

DAIRY-FREE | GLUTEN-FREE | PROTEIN | FIBER | VEGAN

SERVES 2 | PREP TIME: 5 MINUTES | BLEND TIME: <1 MINUTE

Raspberries, blackberries, and cherries are deep-colored fruits, rich in anti-inflammatory phytonutrients. They are also lower-glycemic-index fruits, meaning they have less of an impact on your blood sugar. This smoothie is a great source of fiber.

1 cup frozen berry
  blend (raspberry/
  blackberry/cherry)
½ banana

1 cup organic,
  unsweetened vanilla
  soy milk
3 large ice cubes

1. Put berry blend, banana, soy milk, and ice cubes into the blender.

2. Cover and blend until smooth and creamy.

3. Serve and enjoy immediately.

SUBSTITUTION TIP: Want to add a serving of vegetables to your day? Add one handful of spinach to this smoothie before blending.

Per serving: Calories: 103/Total fat: 2g/Carbohydrates: 17g/Fiber: 3g/Protein: 4g

Golden Tonic Smoothie

DAIRY-FREE | GLUTEN-FREE | LOW-CALORIE | FIBER | VEGAN

SERVES 2 | PREP TIME: 5 MINUTES | BLEND TIME: <1 MINUTE

Turmeric is an anti-inflammatory treasure—it will turn your smoothies or dishes to gold. Sweet mango and banana pair perfectly with this aromatic root.

1 cup frozen
  mango chunks
½ banana

½ teaspoon
  turmeric powder

1 cup organic,
  unsweetened vanilla
  almond milk
3 large ice cubes

1. Put the mango chunks, banana, turmeric powder, almond milk, and ice cubes into the blender.

2. Cover and blend until smooth and creamy.

3. Serve and enjoy immediately.

SUBSTITUTION TIP: Add fresh grated ginger for a little spice.

Per serving: Calories: 97/Total fat: 2g/Carbohydrates: 21g/Fiber: 3g/Protein: 2g

Green Goodness Smoothie

DAIRY-FREE | GLUTEN-FREE | HEALTHY FAT | VEGAN

SERVES 2 | PREP TIME: 5 MINUTES, PLUS OVERNIGHT TO SOAK | BLEND TIME: <1 MINUTE

The spinach and mango in this smoothie provide a good dose of vitamin A, which supports immune health. It also has a good amount of calcium and vitamin C.

½ cup almonds

1 apple, chopped

1 cup spinach

½ cup frozen
 mango chunks

¾ cup water

1 teaspoon matcha for an
 uplifting start to the day
 (optional)

1. Soak the almonds in water overnight. Be sure the almonds are covered before you place them in the refrigerator.

2. Chop the apple into chunks.

3. Put the almonds, apple, spinach, mango, water, and matcha (if using) into the blender.

4. Cover and blend until smooth and creamy.

5. Serve and enjoy immediately.

SUBSTITUTION TIP: Use unpeeled apple for a dose of insoluble fiber.

Per serving: Calories: 290/Total fat: 10g/Carbohydrates: 35g/Fiber: 5g/Protein: 15g

Piña Kale-ada Smoothie

PROBIOTICS | GLUTEN-FREE | HIGH-PROTEIN | HIGH-FIBER | VEGETARIAN

SERVES 2 | PREP TIME: 5 MINUTES | BLEND TIME: <1 MINUTE

Drinking your vegetables in the morning is a great way to sneak in an extra serving of them, and this smoothie includes a dose of vitamin K and phytonutrient-rich kale. Fermented foods such as yogurt are a great source of probiotics. Coconut extract can be found in most grocery stores in the baking aisle near the vanilla.

2 cups curly kale leaves

1 cup frozen
   pineapple chunks

½ banana

1 cup nonfat organic
   Greek yogurt

½ cup nonfat milk or milk
   alternative

2 tablespoons hemp seeds

¼ teaspoon coconut extract

1 teaspoon matcha
   (optional)

1. Rinse the kale and remove the leaves from the stem.

2. Put the kale, pineapple, banana, yogurt, milk, hemp seeds, coconut extract, and matcha (if using) into the blender.

3. Cover and blend until smooth and creamy.

4. Serve and enjoy immediately.

SUBSTITUTION TIP: For a dairy-free option, use a coconut kefir or yogurt to keep probiotics in this smoothie.

Per serving: Calories: 240/Total fat: 5g/Carbohydrates: 35g/Fiber: 6g/Protein: 15g

Berry Refresh Smoothie

DAIRY-FREE | GLUTEN-FREE | HEALTHY FAT | HIGH-FIBER | VEGAN

SERVES 1 | PREP TIME: 5 MINUTES | BLEND TIME: <1 MINUTE

Blueberries are loaded with phytonutrients, and cucumber has a very refreshing flavor. This smoothie is perfect for a summer morning.

1 cup frozen blueberries

½ medium cucumber

2 tablespoons ground flaxseed

1 cup water

3 large ice cubes

4 fresh mint leaves (optional)

1. Put the blueberries, cucumber, flaxseed, water, ice cubes, and mint (if using) into the blender.

2. Cover and blend until smooth and creamy.

3. Serve and enjoy immediately.

NUTRITION TIP: Adding mint increases antioxidant activity. Mint is rich in polyphenols that can reduce oxidative cellular damage.

Per serving: Calories: 160/Total fat: 7g/Carbohydrates: 24g/Fiber: 7g/Protein: 4g

PB&J Smoothie

DAIRY-FREE | GLUTEN-FREE | HIGH-PROTEIN | HIGH-FIBER | VEGAN

SERVES 1 | PREP TIME: 5 MINUTES | BLEND TIME: <1 MINUTE

Nut butters make a good addition to smoothies for a serving of healthy poly-unsaturated fat and a bump of protein.

½ cup frozen strawberries
½ cup frozen blueberries
2 tablespoons
  peanut butter

1 tablespoon ground
  flaxseed

¾ cup organic,
  unsweetened vanilla
  almond milk

1. Put the strawberries, blueberries, peanut butter, flaxseed, and almond milk into the blender.

2. Cover and blend until smooth and creamy.

3. Serve and enjoy immediately.

NUTRITION TIP: The ground flaxseed provides a good serving of fiber to help with bowel regularity.

Per serving: Calories: 310/Total fat: 22g/Carbohydrates: 25g/Fiber: 8g/Protein: 11g

Creamy Chocolate-Berry Smoothie

DAIRY-FREE | GLUTEN-FREE | HEALTHY FAT | HIGH-FIBER | VEGAN

SERVES 1 | PREP TIME: 5 MINUTES | BLEND TIME: <1 MINUTE

Not only does silken tofu add creamy protein to a smoothie, but it's also a source of isoflavones, which are anti-inflammatory phytonutrients.

4 ounces silken tofu

¼ cup frozen
avocado chunks

2 tablespoons
cocoa powder

½ cup frozen berries

2 teaspoons real
maple syrup

¾ cup organic,
unsweetened vanilla
almond milk

3 large ice cubes

1. Put the tofu, avocado, cocoa powder, berries, maple syrup, almond milk, and ice cubes into the blender.

2. Cover and blend until smooth and creamy.

3. Serve and enjoy immediately.

SUBSTITUTION TIP: Make it double chocolate by using unsweetened chocolate almond milk.

Per serving: Calories: 275/Total fat: 15g/Carbohydrates: 30g/Fiber: 10g/Protein: 10g

Make-Ahead Farmers'-Market-Finds Frittata

GLUTEN-FREE | HIGH-PROTEIN | VEGETARIAN

SERVES 8 | PREP TIME: 10 MINUTES | COOK TIME: 30 MINUTES

This recipe includes specific vegetables, but you also can substitute 5 cups of any vegetables you find in-season at your farmers' market. Leftovers can be stored in the refrigerator for 3 to 4 days or frozen for a quick breakfast later. Enjoy with a slice of whole-grain or gluten-free bread.

1 tablespoon extra-virgin olive oil

10 large eggs

2 to 3 tablespoons milk or water

2 cups mozzarella, shredded

1 tablespoon oregano, basil, or other herbs of your choice

½ medium yellow onion, chopped

3 cups fresh spinach

1 cup mushrooms, chopped

1 cup bell pepper, sliced

1. Preheat the oven to 350°F and coat a 9-by-12 baking dish with olive oil.

2. In a bowl, whisk the eggs and milk or water.

3. Add the shredded cheese and herbs and mix well.

4. Fold in the vegetables.

5. Pour the mixture into the baking dish and bake for 30 minutes, or until lightly browned on top.

MAKE IT EASY: Using prechopped or frozen vegetables will cut down on time standing to prepare the meal. If you are using frozen spinach, be sure to squeeze out excess water.

Per serving: Calories: 129/Total fat: 9g/Carbohydrates: 3g/Fiber: 1g/Protein: 10g

Cinnamon-Peach Overnight Oats

GLUTEN-FREE | HEALTHY FAT | HIGH-PROTEIN | HIGH-FIBER | VEGETARIAN

SERVES 2 | PREP TIME: 5 MINUTES, THEN OVERNIGHT

This hearty, whole-grain breakfast can be eaten cold. Using baking spices such as cinnamon is a great way to add perceived sweetness without loading on the sugar.

1 cup plain low-fat yogurt
2 teaspoons maple syrup
½ teaspoon cinnamon

1 cup old-fashioned
   rolled oats

1 cup frozen or fresh
   peach slices
½ cup walnuts, divided

1. In a medium bowl, stir the yogurt, maple syrup, and cinnamon until well combined.

2. Add the oats and stir until well combined.

3. Stir in the fruit and cover.

4. Place in refrigerator overnight and enjoy the following morning topped with ¼ cup walnuts.

NUTRITION TIP: Including yogurt in your diet provides a source of probiotics that can help balance your microbiome.

Per serving: Calories: 465/Total fat: 25g/Carbohydrates: 51g/Fiber: 7g/Protein: 17g

Berry-licious Overnight Oats

SERVES 2 | PREP TIME: 5 MINUTES, THEN OVERNIGHT

This recipe takes 5 minutes or less of preparation, and the flavor-melding magic happens overnight while you're getting regenerative rest. Prepare in mason jars for a grab-and-go option.

⅔ cup old-fashioned rolled oats

¼ teaspoon ground cinnamon

1⅓ cup 1-percent plain kefir

¼ teaspoon vanilla extract or powder

1½ cups frozen mixed berries

⅛ cup unsweetened coconut flakes

¼ cup nuts (I like almonds in this but you can use walnuts, too)

1. In a large bowl, mix the rolled oats and cinnamon, then add in the kefir and vanilla and mix well.

2. Top with berries and coconut flakes.

3. Cover your bowl and place in the refrigerator overnight or, if you are taking your breakfast to go in the morning, divide the mixture into two storage containers.

4. In the morning, top with nuts and enjoy.

NUTRITION TIP: This breakfast provides prebiotics from the oats and probiotics from the kefir.

Per serving: Calories: 280/Total fat: 9g/Carbohydrates: 45g/Fiber: 8g/Protein: 15g

Spiced Pumpkin Oatmeal

DAIRY-FREE | GLUTEN-FREE OPTION | HEALTHY FAT | HIGH-FIBER | VEGAN

SERVES 1 | PREP TIME: 5 MINUTES | COOK TIME: 3 MINUTES

A quick way to make old-fashioned oats with limited cleanup, this breakfast also provides a dose of immune-supporting vitamin A.

⅓ cup old-fashioned rolled oats

¼ teaspoon pumpkin pie spice or cinnamon

⅓ cup organic, unsweetened almond milk

½ cup pumpkin purée

2 tablespoons dried cherries

1 teaspoon maple syrup

2 tablespoons pumpkin seeds

1. In a medium microwave-safe bowl, stir together the oats and pumpkin pie spice.

2. Add the almond milk, pumpkin purée, cherries, and maple syrup. Stir to combine.

3. Microwave on medium-high for 3 minutes (watching to ensure the oats do not boil over and make a mess).

4. Let stand in microwave for 5 minutes.

5. Top with pumpkin seeds and enjoy warm.

SUBSTITUTION TIP: If you do not tolerate seeds well or have difficulty chewing, add a tablespoon of sunflower butter instead.

Per serving: Calories: 246/Total fat: 4g/Carbohydrates: 49g/Fiber: 10g/Protein: 7g

Salmon-Avocado Toast

GLUTEN-FREE OPTION | HEALTHY FAT | PROTEIN | HIGH-FIBER

SERVES 1 | PREP TIME: 10 MINUTES

This recipe can be made with leftover salmon or you can use smoked salmon that comes ready to eat. Use gluten-free or another whole-grain bread, and choose 100 percent whole-grain for the fiber.

1 slice whole-grain bread
½ avocado
2 ounces salmon

3 or 4 cherry
   tomatoes, halved
Basil, dried or
   chopped fresh

Turmeric
Freshly ground
   black pepper

1. Toast the bread to the desired crispness.

2. Mash the avocado on the toast and spread evenly.

3. Flake the salmon on top of the avocado, and top with the tomato halves.

4. Season to your preference with basil, pepper, and turmeric.

SUBSTITUTION TIP: As a bread-free alternative, you can make a savory breakfast bowl. Use millet or quinoa as a base and top with the remaining ingredients.

Per serving: Calories: 220/Total fat: 11g/Carbohydrates: 25g/Fiber: 8g/Protein: 6g

Southwest Tofu Scramble

DAIRY-FREE | GLUTEN-FREE | HIGH-PROTEIN | HIGH-FIBER | VEGAN

SERVES 2 | PREP TIME: 10 MINUTES | COOK TIME: 10 MINUTES

Tofu is a great egg substitute, especially for anyone with an egg intolerance, and offers another way to use a plant-based food that provides phytonutrients.

8 ounces extra-firm tofu

1 to 2 tablespoons extra-virgin olive oil

1 cup frozen onion-and-bell-pepper blend

¼ teaspoon turmeric

¼ teaspoon garlic powder

¼ teaspoon paprika

1 handful spinach or kale

½ cup black beans

4 tablespoons salsa

1. Cover the tofu with paper towels and place a heavy pan on top to drain the excess liquid.

2. Mash the tofu with a potato masher or fork into chunks.

3. In a medium sauté pan or skillet, heat the oil over medium heat and sauté the onions and peppers for 3 minutes.

4. Add the tofu and scramble for 1 minute.

5. Mix the turmeric, garlic powder, and paprika and sprinkle evenly over the tofu scramble.

6. Continue to scramble for about 2 minutes, and then add the spinach and black beans.

7. Cook for about 2 minutes, or until the spinach is slightly wilted. Remove from the heat and enjoy topped with salsa.

SUBSTITUTION TIP: Use fresh chopped vegetables if you can. I am using frozen here to make the recipe easier for anyone who feels like a shortcut is in order.

Per serving: Calories: 310/Total fat: 8g/Carbohydrates: 35g/Fiber: 10g/Protein: 23g

Easy Breakfast Hash

DAIRY-FREE | GLUTEN-FREE | HIGH-PROTEIN | HIGH-FIBER | VEGETARIAN

SERVES 2 | PREP TIME: 10 MINUTES | COOK TIME: 10 MINUTES

Sweet potatoes are an excellent source of important nutrients, such as potassium, fiber, and vitamin C. They also provide smaller amounts of thiamin, B_6, iron, and magnesium.

1 medium sweet potato

1 tablespoon extra-virgin olive oil

¼ teaspoon garlic powder

¼ teaspoon rosemary

3 eggs

1 cup kale, chopped

Salt

Freshly ground black pepper

1. Scrub the sweet potato and pierce it several times with a fork. Microwave it for 3 minutes, turn it over, and microwave it for 2 more minutes.

2. Heat the oil in a medium nonstick pan over medium heat while the sweet potato is cooling.

3. Chop the sweet potato into cubes and add to the pan along with the garlic powder and rosemary.

4. Sauté for 3 minutes, allowing the sweet potato to brown slightly.

5. While the sweet potato continues to cook, whisk the eggs.

6. Add the kale and stir until slightly wilted.

7. Add the eggs to the pan and scramble with the hash mixture. Add salt and pepper to taste.

8. Once the eggs are cooked, plate and enjoy right away.

NUTRITION TIP: Vitamin C helps you absorb iron from plant sources.

Per serving: Calories: 369/Total fat: 12g/Carbohydrates: 49g/Fiber: 6g/Protein: 17g

Savory Quinoa Breakfast Bowl

DAIRY-FREE | GLUTEN-FREE | HIGH-PROTEIN | HIGH-FIBER | VEGETARIAN

SERVES 1 | PREP TIME: 10 MINUTES | COOK TIME: 5 MINUTES

Leftover quinoa makes a great base for a breakfast bowl. While toast, pancakes, and waffles are traditional breakfast foods, this whole grain is higher in fiber and a complete protein.

1 tablespoon extra-virgin olive oil

½ cup frozen onion-and-bell-pepper blend

½ cup mushrooms

½ cup cooked quinoa

1 tablespoon pesto

1 egg

Salt

Freshly ground black pepper

1 tablespoon feta cheese, crumbled (optional)

1. In a small sauté pan, heat the oil over medium heat.

2. Sauté the frozen onions and peppers with the mushrooms until soft, about 4 minutes; set aside.

3. Microwave the leftover quinoa, then stir in the pesto.

4. Distribute the cooked vegetables over the quinoa and cover to keep warm.

5. Using the same pan, fry the egg and place it on top of the quinoa bowl.

6. Season with salt and pepper, sprinkle with feta cheese (if using), and enjoy.

SUBSTITUTION TIP: You can swap in tofu in place of the egg if you do not tolerate eggs well.

Per serving: Calories: 400/Total fat: 12g/Carbohydrates: 55g/Fiber: 6g/Protein: 19g

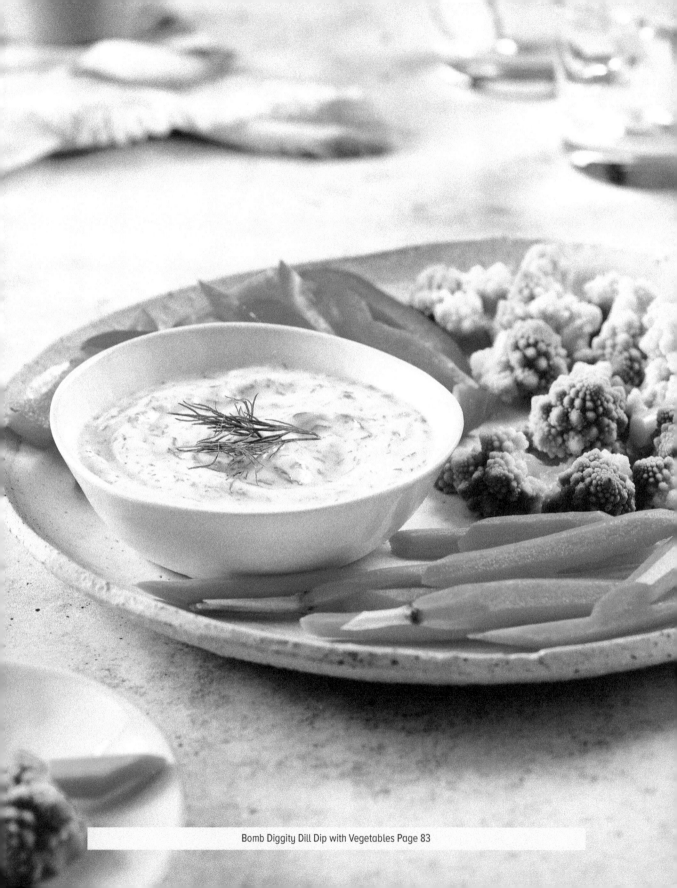

Bomb Diggity Dill Dip with Vegetables Page 83

CHAPTER FIVE

Snacks
and Sides

Nut- or Seed-Butter Celery Boats

DAIRY-FREE | GLUTEN-FREE | NUT-FREE OPTION | VEGAN

SERVES 1 | PREP TIME: 2 MINUTES

Healthy fat, fiber, phytonutrients, and protein are all included in this simple, no-cook snack.

2 to 3 celery stalks

2 tablespoons nut or seed butter

2 tablespoons dried blueberries or cherries

1. Wash the celery and cut it into 2- to 3-inch pieces, discarding the white ends and the leaves on top.

2. Using a spoon or knife, fill the celery bed with the nut or seed butter of your choice.

3. Top with dried blueberries or cherries.

MAKE IT EASY: Cut all your celery at once so the snack is easy to throw together when you don't have time or energy.

Per serving: Calories: 295/Total fat: 17g/Carbohydrates: 37g/Fiber: 6g/Protein: 10g

Freestyle Snack to Go

DAIRY-FREE | GLUTEN-FREE | NUT-FREE-OPTION | VEGAN

SERVES 1 | PREP TIME: 2 MINUTES

Having foods ready to grab and go can set you up for healthy snacking when hunger hits. This freestyle snack is a simple, balanced option that can provide you the fuel you need to get you from breakfast to lunch.

1 small banana, 1 medium orange, 1 pear, or ½ cup raspberries, blackberries, or cherries

¼ cup almonds, pecans, walnuts, pumpkin seeds, and/or sunflower seeds

1. Wash the fruit (if it doesn't have skin or a peel).

2. Enjoy.

NUTRITION TIP: Do not prewash your berries, which increases the potential for harmful bacteria to grow. Wash fruit just before eating or packing for the day.

Per serving varies based on choices. Per serving with 1 small banana and ¼ cup almonds: Calories: 294/Total fat: 18g/Carbohydrates: 31g/Fiber: 7g/Protein: 9g

Crisp Roasted Chickpeas

DAIRY-FREE | GLUTEN-FREE | HIGH-PROTEIN | HIGH-FIBER | VEGAN

SERVES 4 | PREP TIME: 5 MINUTES | COOK TIME: 30 MINUTES

These delicious crisp beans make a balanced snack on their own. They provide protein, carbohydrates, and fiber, and the olive oil adds healthy monounsaturated fat. Instead of the spices listed, you can use curry powder if you have it on hand to save time.

2 teaspoons turmeric

1 teaspoon cumin

1 teaspoon paprika

2 (15-ounce) cans chickpeas, rinsed, drained, and patted dry

¼ teaspoon freshly ground black pepper

1 tablespoon extra-virgin olive oil

1. Preheat the oven to 350°F.

2. Line 2 baking sheets with parchment paper.

3. In a small bowl, stir the turmeric, cumin, paprika, and pepper to combine.

4. Spread the chickpeas on the baking sheets in a single layer, sprinkle with the seasoning blend, and drizzle with olive oil. Lightly toss with your hands to evenly coat the chickpeas.

5. Bake for 30 to 40 minutes until nicely browned and lightly crisp.

MAKE IT EASY: These can be used to add crunch and spice—as well as a boost of fiber and protein—to a salad or vegetable entrée.

Per serving: Calories: 220/Total fat: 5g/Carbohydrates: 35g/Fiber: 12g/Protein: 12g

Bomb Diggity Dill Dip
with Vegetables

DAIRY-FREE | GLUTEN-FREE | PROTEIN | FIBER | VEGAN

SERVES 8 | PREP TIME: 6 MINUTES

This dip is so light and fluffy it can even be served with softer cooked vegetables. It's also versatile enough to be used as a salad dressing.

6 ounces organic
  silken tofu
3 tablespoons fresh dill
1 garlic clove
1½ tablespoons lemon juice

½ teaspoon onion powder
Salt
Freshly ground
  black pepper

1 teaspoon nutritional yeast
  (optional)
½ cup carrots, sliced
½ red bell pepper, sliced

1. Add the tofu, dill, garlic, lemon juice, onion powder, salt and pepper to taste, and nutritional yeast (if using) to a food processor or blender.

2. Cover and blend until smooth and creamy.

3. Chill in the refrigerator for 1 hour or more before serving with carrots and bell pepper.

MAKE IT EASY: This dip can be stored in an airtight container for up to 3 days.

Per serving: Calories: 94/Total fat: 2g/Carbohydrates: 12g/Fiber: 4g/Protein: 4g

Beet and Goat Cheese Tartines

WHOLE GRAIN | FIBER | ANTIOXIDANT | VEGETARIAN

SERVES 1 | PREP TIME: 5 MINUTES | COOK TIME: 5 MINUTES (35 MINUTES IF ROASTING BEETS)

Beets are loaded with antioxidant, anti-inflammatory, and detox-supporting nutrients. They also contain betaine, a neuroprotectant.

1 slice whole-wheat bread, lightly toasted

2 small cooked beets

1 ounce goat cheese

Small handful arugula

1 tablespoon tarragon or herb of your choice

Salt

Freshly ground black pepper

1. Cut the toast and beets into quarters.

2. Spread the goat cheese evenly over the toast quarters.

3. Top the goat cheese with the arugula and the beets.

4. Sprinkle with the tarragon, salt, and pepper.

MAKE IT EASY: If you have the time, you can roast the beets yourself. Cut them into smaller pieces before roasting to cut down on time in the oven. Toss with olive oil, salt, and pepper and roast for 30 minutes at 425°F.

Per serving: Calories: 198/Total fat: 7g/Carbohydrates: 24g/Fiber: 4g/Protein: 10g

Garlic Cauliflower Mash

DAIRY-FREE OPTION | GLUTEN-FREE | LOW-CARB | FIBER | VEGETARIAN

SERVES 4 | PREP TIME: 10 MINUTES | COOK TIME: 5 MINUTES

Cauliflower may be white, but don't let that fool you. It is still loaded with just as many phytonutrients as other colorful, sulfur-rich vegetables.

1 cauliflower head, cut into florets

1 or 2 garlic cloves, smashed

2 tablespoons extra-virgin olive oil

¼ cup milk or milk alternative

Salt

Freshly ground black pepper

Rosemary, for garnish

1. Fill a medium pan with ¼ inch of water and bring to a boil.

2. Add the cauliflower, cover, and cook until soft, about 5 minutes. Remove from heat and drain. (You can microwave frozen cauliflower to reduce time and cleanup.)

3. While the cauliflower cooks, sauté the garlic in olive oil over medium heat until fragrant and soft, about 2 minutes.

4. Add the cauliflower, garlic, milk, and salt and pepper to taste to a food processor or blender and purée until smooth.

5. Serve warm, sprinkled with rosemary.

NUTRITION TIP: Reduce the total carbohydrates in any meal by using cauliflower mash instead of mashed potatoes.

Per serving: Calories: 127/Total fat: 7g/Carbohydrates: 13g/Fiber: 5g/Protein: 5g

Zesty Roasted Broccoli

GLUTEN-FREE | HEALTHY FAT | HIGH-FIBER

SERVES 6 TO 8 | PREP TIME: 5 MINUTES | COOK TIME: 25 MINUTES

Broccoli is a brain-boosting vegetable that tastes fabulous roasted. Lemon zest and Parmesan add a bit of zest and savory notes.

2 large broccoli heads, cut into large florets

3 tablespoons extra-virgin olive oil

1 tablespoon grated Parmesan cheese

1 teaspoon lemon zest

Salt

Freshly ground black pepper

1. Preheat the oven to 450°F.

2. Toss the broccoli in the oil on a baking sheet.

3. Roast, tossing occasionally until slightly browned, about 25 minutes.

4. Sprinkle with the Parmesan cheese and lemon zest, and season with salt and pepper.

SUBSTITUTION TIP: Use nutritional yeast in place of Parmesan for a delicious, dairy-free alternative.

Per serving: Calories: 80/Total fat: 5g/Carbohydrates: 13g/Fiber: 5g/Protein: 6g

Shiitake Mushroom Wild Rice

DAIRY-FREE | GLUTEN-FREE | PROTEIN | HIGH-FIBER

SERVES 6 | PREP TIME: 20 MINUTES | COOK TIME: 45 MINUTES

Shiitake mushrooms are a good source of some B vitamins, antioxidants, and anti-inflammatory compounds. The shiitake mushrooms in this recipe give the wild rice immune-supporting properties.

2 cups low-sodium chicken or vegetable broth
2 cups sliced shiitake mushrooms
1 cup wild or brown rice

1 teaspoon avocado oil
1 bunch scallions, trimmed and sliced
6 tablespoons whole or sliced almonds

Salt
Freshly ground black pepper

1. In a medium saucepan, bring the broth to boil over high heat.

2. Stir in the mushrooms and rice and allow to boil.

3. Reduce the heat to low, cover, and simmer for about 45 minutes.

4. About 5 minutes before the rice is done, heat the oil over medium heat in a medium pan. Add the scallions and cook, stirring frequently, for 2 to 3 minutes.

5. Drain any excess liquid from the rice and mix with the scallions and almonds in a serving bowl. Stir to combine, and season with salt and pepper.

MAKE IT EASY: If using whole almonds, lightly chop before adding into the dish.

Per serving: Calories: 150/Total fat: 4g/Carbohydrates: 24g/Fiber: 5g/Protein: 6g

Baked Sweet Potato Wedges

DAIRY-FREE | GLUTEN-FREE | HIGH-FIBER | VEGAN

SERVES 6 | PREP TIME: 5 MINUTES | COOK TIME: 35 MINUTES

These sweet potato wedges can replace fries as a side or be served as a quick snack. Sweet potatoes are loaded with nutrients and fiber. Rosemary also has anti-inflammatory properties.

2 pounds sweet potatoes
2 to 3 tablespoons
  extra-virgin olive oil

2 tablespoons fresh
  rosemary, chopped
Salt

Freshly ground
  black pepper

1. Preheat the oven to 450°F.

2. Cut the sweet potatoes in half lengthwise, then cut each half into 4 to 5 wedges.

3. Place the wedges on a baking sheet and toss with olive oil, rosemary, and salt and pepper.

4. Arrange the potatoes in a single layer and roast until they are golden brown, 20 to 25 minutes.

5. Enjoy hot.

SUBSTITUTION TIP: For a treat that's both sweet and savory, sprinkle with cinnamon.

Per serving: Calories: 144/Total fat: 4g/Carbohydrates: 30g/Fiber: 5g/Protein: 2g

Brussels Sprouts

DAIRY-FREE | GLUTEN-FREE | SULFUR-RICH | FIBER

SERVES 4 | PREP TIME: 10 MINUTES | COOK TIME: 20 MINUTES

Brussels sprouts are loaded with phytonutrients, vitamin K, vitamin C, B vitamins, and fiber. These nutrient-dense vegetables promote detox pathways, fight free radicals, and provide immune support. They are a wonderfully tasty side with a hint of mustard flavor.

2 cups Brussels sprouts

1½ tablespoons extra-virgin olive oil

1½ tablespoons balsamic vinegar

1 tablespoon minced garlic

1 teaspoon turmeric

Salt

Freshly ground black pepper

1. Preheat oven to 450°F and line a baking sheet with parchment paper.

2. Rinse the Brussels sprouts, chop off the stem ends, and halve.

3. Whisk the oil, vinegar, garlic, turmeric, and salt and pepper to taste. Drizzle over the sprouts and toss to combine.

4. Spread the sprouts evenly over the baking sheet and bake for 20 to 25 minutes.

5. Enjoy warm.

NUTRITION TIP: Sulfur-rich vegetables are an important part of a well-balanced diet. If you don't like Brussels sprouts, try roasting a serving of broccoli, cauliflower, or turnips.

Per serving: Calories: 72/Total fat: 5g/Carbohydrates: 6g/Fiber: 2g/Protein: 2g

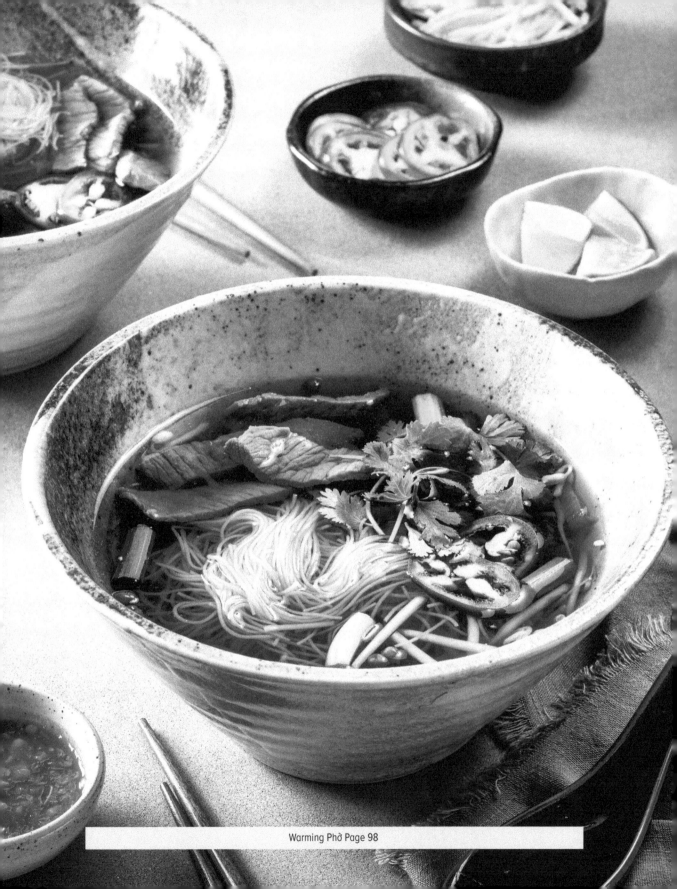

CHAPTER SIX

Soups, Stews, and Broths

Vegetable Broth

DAIRY-FREE | GLUTEN-FREE | LOW-CALORIE | VEGAN

SERVES 10 | PREP TIME: 10 MINUTES | COOK TIME: 2 HOURS

The seaweed in this broth is a great source of omega-3 fatty acids, iron, magnesium, calcium, and iodine. It also provides umami—a rich, savory, and comforting flavor.

12 cups filtered water

2 cups kale or collard greens, chopped

2 sheets dried kombu seaweed

4 medium carrots, coarsely chopped

2 medium onions, quartered

½ bunch celery stalks, coarsely chopped

6 dried shiitake mushrooms

6 garlic cloves, smashed

1 bunch thyme, cilantro, or parsley

1 teaspoon black peppercorns

1 (2-inch) piece ginger, sliced (optional)

1. Combine the water, kale, seaweed, carrots, onions, celery stalks, mushrooms, garlic, thyme, peppercorns, and ginger (if using) in a large stockpot or slow cooker. Bring to a boil, then cover and simmer for 2 hours.

2. Add more water if it evaporates during cooking and the vegetables are exposed.

3. Strain the vegetables from the broth and discard. Cool and store in the refrigerator or freezer for later use.

MAKE IT EASY: When storing in the freezer, use large, silicone ice cube trays. This makes the broth easier to defrost when you want to use it for a recipe or enjoy a cup of broth.

Per serving: Calories: 60/Total fat: 0g/Carbohydrates: 14g/Fiber: 1g/Protein: 1g

Easy Beans 'n' Greens

DAIRY-FREE | GLUTEN-FREE | HIGH-FIBER | BONE SUPPORT | VEGAN OPTION

SERVES 5 | PREP TIME: 10 MINUTES | COOK TIME: 15 MINUTES

Support your gut, bone, and immune health with this fiber-rich soup that also has more than 100 percent of your daily value of calcium and vitamin A and a good dose of vitamin C and iron.

2 tablespoons extra-virgin olive oil

1 large onion, chopped

3 garlic cloves, sliced

¼ teaspoon red pepper flakes

Salt

Freshly ground black pepper

4 cups kale, collard greens, or escarole, chopped

2 (15-ounce) cans cannellini beans, drained and rinsed

2 cups low-sodium or homemade broth

1. In a large stockpot, heat the oil over medium heat and sauté the onion and garlic for about 3 minutes, or until tender.

2. Add the red pepper flakes, and salt and pepper to taste and sauté until fragrant. Add the greens and sauté for about 3 minutes, or until tender.

3. Add the beans and broth, cover, and cook for 15 to 20 minutes.

SUBSTITUTION TIP: Add a can of diced tomatoes for an alternative way to enjoy this soup.

Per serving: Calories: 238/Total fat: 7g/Carbohydrates: 33g/Fiber: 10g/Protein: 12g

Hearty Sweet Potato and Kale Soup

DAIRY-FREE | GLUTEN-FREE | HIGH-FIBER | VEGAN OPTION

SERVES 8 | PREP TIME: 10 MINUTES | COOK TIME: 5 TO 8 HOURS

This colorful soup is loaded with fiber, vitamins, and minerals that support detoxification processes in the body and immune function.

2 sweet potatoes, peeled and cubed

2 cups carrots, peeled and diced

5 celery stalks, chopped

1 cup split peas

1 cup green lentils

1 medium yellow onion, chopped

5 garlic cloves, minced

10 cups low-sodium broth

1 teaspoon cumin

1 teaspoon freshly ground black pepper

½ cup extra-virgin olive oil (infused is okay)

4 cups kale, chopped

1 cup parsley, chopped

1 tablespoon lemon juice

1. Combine the sweet potatoes, carrots, celery, split peas, lentils, onion, garlic, broth, cumin, and pepper in a slow cooker or large stockpot.

2. If using a slow cooker, cook on high heat for 5 to 6 hours or on low heat for 7 to 8 hours. If using a stockpot, cover and cook over medium to medium-low heat for 5 to 6 hours. The peas and lentils should be soft.

3. Pulse about 4 cups of the finished soup in a blender with the olive oil until creamy but not completely smooth.

4. Add the kale, parsley, and blended soup to the pot and stir to combine over low heat. Add the lemon juice, stir, and cover. Remove from the heat and allow the flavors to blend for 5 to 10 minutes before serving.

SUBSTITUTION TIP: Use cooked split peas and lentils to make this soup in under 30 minutes.

Per serving: Calories: 342/Total fat: 17g/Carbohydrates: 37g/Fiber: 14g/Protein: 17g

Creamy Tomato-Basil Soup

DAIRY-FREE | GLUTEN-FREE | VEGAN OPTION

SERVES 8 | PREP TIME: 10 MINUTES | COOK TIME: 30 MINUTES

The blended cashews in this soup add rich texture and flavor and provide more protein than the cream used in traditional creamy tomato soups.

1 cup cashews

½ cup water

¼ cup extra-virgin olive oil

1 yellow onion, chopped

4 to 6 garlic cloves, minced

1 (28-ounce) can whole, peeled tomatoes

4 cups low-sodium broth

½ cup fresh basil

½ teaspoon oregano

Salt

Freshly ground black pepper

1. In a shallow bowl, combine the cashews and water. Allow the nuts to soak for at least 20 minutes.

2. Meanwhile, in a medium saucepan or high-sided skillet, heat the olive oil over medium heat. Sauté the onions for about 3 minutes or until translucent, then add the garlic, cooking for about 2 minutes or until fragrant. Add the tomatoes, breaking them up with a spoon or spatula while they cook.

3. Add the broth, cover, and simmer for 20 minutes. Add the basil and leave on heat for another 5 minutes.

4. In a blender, blend the cashews and water until smooth and creamy. Transfer the cashew cream to a small bowl and set aside.

5. Blend the soup in the blender in batches until creamy.

6. Return the soup to the pot and bring to a simmer.

7. Whisk in the cashew cream, and season with oregano and salt and pepper to taste. Serve hot.

MAKE IT EASY: Instead of soaking the cashews, use ¼ to ½ cup cashew butter, depending on how rich you want your soup to be.

Per serving: Calories: 196/Total fat: 15g/Carbohydrates: 13g/Fiber: 2g/Protein: 4g

Curry Carrot Soup

DAIRY-FREE | GLUTEN-FREE | VEGAN OPTION

SERVES 6 | PREP TIME: 10 MINUTES | COOK TIME: 25 MINUTES

Fat-soluble vitamins A and K are the superstars of this recipe, and the fat content from the coconut milk and pepitas will help you absorb all the beneficial fat-soluble vitamins.

1 large onion, chopped

3 cups low-sodium broth, divided

4 garlic cloves, chopped

2 tablespoons fresh ginger, grated

1 to 2 teaspoons curry powder

2 cups carrots, chopped about ½-inch thick

2 cups sweet potato, chopped about ½-inch thick

1 can light coconut milk

Salt

Freshly ground black pepper

⅓ cup pepitas

1. In a medium to large soup pot, sauté the onion in 1 tablespoon of broth for about 3 minutes, or until soft.

2. Add the garlic and ginger and sauté for about 1 minute, or until fragrant. Add the curry powder and stir well to combine.

3. Add the remaining broth, carrots, and sweet potatoes, and simmer over medium heat for 20 minutes, or until the vegetables are tender. Add the coconut milk and stir to combine.

4. Blend the soup in batches in a blender or food processor until creamy, or use an immersion blender. Keep in mind that hot contents in a blender can increase the pressure, causing the soup to splash out when you open it.

5. Once all of the soup is blended, return it to the pot, add salt and pepper to taste, and reheat before serving.

6. Top each serving with 1 tablespoon of pepitas.

SUBSTITUTION TIP: If you prefer to skip the crunchy topping, you can top with fresh herbs of your choice.

Per serving: Calories: 185/Total fat: 8g/Carbohydrates: 19g/Fiber: 4g/Protein: 7g

Roasted Cauliflower Soup

DAIRY-FREE | GLUTEN-FREE | LOW-FAT | LOW-CALORIE | VEGAN OPTION

SERVES 5 | PREP TIME: 10 MINUTES | COOK TIME: 45 MINUTES

Golden turmeric doesn't only make this soup pop with color—it's full of anti-inflammatory curcumin. Be sure to add black pepper, which increases your body's absorption of the turmeric.

6 cups cauliflower florets (about 1 large head)

4 garlic cloves, coarsely chopped

1 tablespoon extra-virgin olive oil, divided

1 medium yellow onion, diced

1 tablespoon fresh ginger, grated

2 teaspoons turmeric

1 teaspoon cumin

4 cups water or low-sodium broth

1 cup unsweetened, light coconut milk

Salt

Freshly ground black pepper

2 tablespoons lemon juice

2 tablespoons sunflower seeds

5 tablespoons chopped cilantro, microgreens, or herb of your choice

1. Preheat the oven to 450°F. On a baking sheet, drizzle the cauliflower and garlic with about 1 teaspoon of the olive oil. Toss to evenly coat and roast for 25 minutes. Turn the cauliflower halfway through roasting.

2. Meanwhile, heat the remaining olive oil in a medium soup pot over medium heat and cook the onions for about 5 minutes, or until soft. Add the ginger, turmeric, and cumin, mixing well to combine.

3. Add the broth, roasted cauliflower (reserving one cup), and garlic. Bring to a boil, then reduce heat and simmer 10 minutes.

4. Blend the soup in batches, or use an immersion blender if you have one, to blend until creamy.

5. Return the soup to the pot and add the coconut milk, stirring to combine. Season with salt and pepper, add lemon juice, and stir. Serve warm, topped with the reserved cauliflower, sunflower seeds, and cilantro.

MAKE IT EASY: Buy chopped cauliflower to cut down on prep time.

Per serving: Calories: 140/Total fat: 7g/Carbohydrates: 14g/Fiber: 3g/Protein: 5g

Warming Phở

DAIRY-FREE | GLUTEN-FREE | HIGH-PROTEIN | LOW-FAT

SERVES 4 | PREP TIME: 10 MINUTES | COOK TIME: 40 MINUTES

This staple of Vietnamese cuisine is a warm, soothing soup that's wonderful to sip and has anti-inflammatory and antimicrobial properties. It's perfect for winter and warding off a cold.

2 star anise pods, or ¼ teaspoon fennel seeds

8 cups unsalted or low-sodium beef broth

1 large onion, halved and thinly sliced

1 (3-inch) piece ginger, peeled and thinly sliced

4 garlic cloves, chopped

1 jalapeño, sliced

4 scallions, cut into 1-inch pieces

1 cup cilantro leaves, chopped

2 cups bean sprouts

1 tablespoon low-sodium soy sauce

1 teaspoon fish sauce

8 ounces rice or shirataki noodles

12-ounces eye round beef, pork ribs, or king trumpet mushrooms, cut into ⅛-inch-thick slices

4 lime wedges

Sriracha and/or hoisin sauce (optional)

1. In a large stockpot, toast the star anise pods over medium heat for about 2 minutes, or until fragrant.

2. Add the broth, onion, ginger, and garlic. Increase the heat to medium-high and bring to a boil. Reduce the heat to low, cover, and simmer for 30 minutes.

3. While the soup simmers, slice the jalapeño, cut the scallions, chop the cilantro, and divide the rinsed bean sprouts among the bowls.

4. When the soup is finished simmering, remove the star anise pods and stir in the soy sauce and fish sauce.

5. Prepare the noodles according to the package directions. Once the noodles have started to cook, add the sliced beef to the soup and cook for 3 minutes.

6. Divide the cooked noodles and bean sprouts among 4 bowls. Ladle the soup over the noodles and bean sprouts.

7. Top with scallions, jalapeños, cilantro, and a squeeze of lime. Add the sriracha and hoisin sauce (if using) or use for dipping.

MAKE IT EASY: Freeze the beef or pork for 1 hour before preparing to make it easier to slice thinly.

Per serving: Calories: 306/Total fat: 7g/Carbohydrates: 26g/Fiber: 3g/Protein: 33g

Simple Miso Soup

DAIRY-FREE | GLUTEN-FREE | FIBER | LOW-CALORIE | VEGAN OPTION

SERVES 4 | PREP TIME: 10 MINUTES | COOK TIME: 12 MINUTES

This soup can be made in just a few minutes by mixing miso and water. Just add your favorite protein and vegetable, such as phytonutrient-rich soybeans, tofu, and spinach.

¼ cup miso paste (red or white)

5 cups water, divided

1 cup frozen shelled edamame

⅛ teaspoon salt

4 cups spinach leaves

1 (16-ounce) package firm tofu, cut into ½-inch cubes

2 scallions, thinly sliced

2 tablespoons sesame seeds

1. In a medium bowl, whisk the miso paste and 1 cup of water.

2. In a medium saucepan, bring the remaining 4 cups of water to a boil and add the edamame and salt. Cook until tender, or about 5 minutes.

3. Stir in the spinach and tofu. Give the miso mixture a stir before adding it to the soup. Add the scallions and stir to combine.

4. Divide the soup among 4 bowls and top with sesame seeds.

MAKE IT EASY: You can buy premade miso soup and just add protein and the vegetables of your choice.

Per serving: Calories: 170/Total fat: 9g/Carbohydrates: 10g/Fiber: 4g/Protein: 15g

Italian Fish Stew

DAIRY-FREE | GLUTEN-FREE | HIGH-PROTEIN | LOW-CALORIE

SERVES 4 | PREP TIME: 10 MINUTES | COOK TIME: 35 MINUTES

Enjoy your favorite types of fish in this easy stew, which is ready in under an hour. Stewing tomatoes makes the anti-inflammatory nutrient lycopene more bioavailable.

2 tablespoons extra-virgin olive oil

3 garlic cloves, chopped

Red pepper flakes

1 pound any combination fresh salmon, cod, shrimp, haddock, and/or calamari, chopped

¼ cup dry white wine

¾ cup tomato purée

1 cup tomatoes, diced

1 cup water

1 tablespoon Italian spice blend

Salt

Freshly ground black pepper

2 baked potatoes (optional)

1. In a large soup pot, heat the oil over medium heat and sauté the garlic and red pepper flakes (to taste) for 1 minute, or until fragrant.

2. Add the fish and stir for about 1 minute. Raise the heat to medium-high, add the white wine, and cook for 2 minutes. Add the tomato purée, diced tomatoes, water, Italian spice blend, and salt and pepper to taste.

3. Bring the soup to a boil, then reduce the heat and simmer for 25 minutes. Serve each bowl with ½ baked potato (if using) to make it a hearty meal.

MAKE IT EASY: You can use 3 to 4 teaspoons of minced garlic to cut down on prep time and save your fingers from smelling like garlic.

Per serving: Calories: 210/Total fat: 10g/Carbohydrates: 9g/Fiber: 2g/Protein: 22g

Slow-Cooker Beef Stew

DAIRY-FREE | GLUTEN-FREE | HIGH-PROTEIN | LOW-CALORIE

SERVES 10 | PREP TIME: 10 MINUTES | COOK TIME: 3 TO 4 HOURS

Beef stew does not have to be as thick as gravy. A light dusting of arrowroot powder on the beef before browning and the potatoes in the stew will thicken it just enough.

1 medium yellow onion, chopped

2 cups carrots, chopped

5 celery stalks, chopped

2 medium red potatoes, chopped

2 turnips, chopped

½ cup tomato paste

4 cups low-sodium broth

1 tablespoon Italian spice blend

2 dried bay leaves

2 pounds boneless chuck roast, cubed

Salt

Freshly ground black pepper

1 tablespoon arrowroot powder

2 tablespoons extra-virgin olive oil

3 garlic cloves, chopped

1 cup diced tomatoes

1. In a slow cooker, combine the onion, carrots, celery, red potatoes, turnips, tomato paste, broth, Italian spice blend, and dried bay leaves.

2. In a large bowl, add the chuck roast and season with salt and pepper. Sprinkle with arrowroot powder and toss to coat.

3. In a medium skillet, heat the oil over medium heat. Add the garlic and beef and cook for about 5 minutes, until the beef is just browned on all sides.

4. Add the browned beef, garlic, and tomatoes to the slow cooker and stir to combine. Cook on high heat for 3 to 4 hours. Serve warm.

NUTRITION TIP: Skim the fat from the top of the stew before serving. This will remove some of the saturated fat from the beef.

Per serving: Calories: 328/Total fat: 19g/Carbohydrates: 16g/Fiber: 3g/Protein: 22g

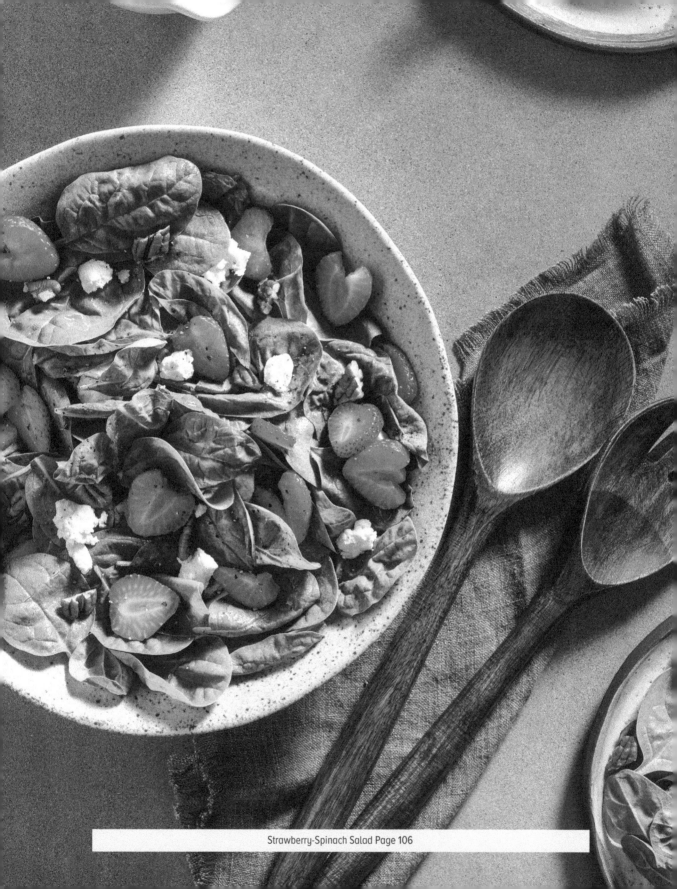

Strawberry-Spinach Salad Page 106

CHAPTER SEVEN

Salads

Strawberry-Spinach Salad

DAIRY-FREE | GLUTEN-FREE OPTION | HEALTHY FAT | HIGH-FIBER | VEGETARIAN

SERVES 2 | PREP TIME: 10 MINUTES

The strawberries complement the spinach perfectly. Not only do they taste great, but they also provide vitamin C, which helps increase iron absorption from the spinach. Having adequate iron intake can help decrease fatigue while providing support to mitochondrial metabolism (energy production) and cellular immune function. This salad also provides a healthy dose of vitamin A and calcium.

2 tablespoons extra-virgin olive oil

1 tablespoon white balsamic vinegar

1 teaspoon maple syrup

Salt

Freshly ground black pepper

1½ cups fresh strawberries, hulled and sliced

4 cups baby spinach

¼ cup pecans, lightly chopped

2 ounces goat cheese, crumbled

1. In a large bowl, whisk the olive oil, vinegar, maple syrup, and salt and pepper to taste.

2. Once everything is mixed well, add the strawberries, spinach, pecans, and goat cheese.

3. Gently toss to coat the with the dressing and serve.

SUBSTITUTION TIP: You can swap the goat cheese for your favorite nut cheese or crumbled tofu. You'll still get the creamy texture, and using tofu will provide more calcium.

Per serving: Calories: 380/Total fat: 32g/Carbohydrates: 20g/Fiber: 7g/Protein: 9g

Cooling Mint-Watermelon Salad

GLUTEN-FREE | LOW-FAT | LOW-CALORIE | VEGETARIAN

SERVES 2 | PREP TIME: 10 MINUTES

The chemical compounds in mint trick your brain into thinking it is cool or cold, when really the temperature in your mouth remains the same. This recipe is a refreshing summer salad that can be enjoyed anytime. Watermelon and blackberries are both phytonutrient-rich fruits with anti-inflammatory and antioxidant properties.

4 cups watermelon, cubed

1 cup blackberries, halved

½ cup crumbled
  feta cheese

½ bunch mint leaves,
  chopped (about 1 cup
  loosely packed)

Juice of ½ lime

Salt, freshly ground black
  pepper, and lime zest
  (optional)

1. In a large bowl, combine the watermelon, blackberries, feta cheese, mint, lime juice, and salt, pepper, and lime zest to taste (if using).

2. Gently toss and serve.

NUTRITION TIP: Cut fruit can retain nutrients up to 6 days if chilled in the refrigerator, so continue to enjoy this salad for almost a week.

Per serving: Calories: 241/Total fat: 8g/Carbohydrates: 38g/Fiber: 10g/Protein: 9g

Superfood Salad

DAIRY-FREE OPTION | GLUTEN-FREE | HEALTHY FAT | HIGH-FIBER

SERVES 4 TO 6 | PREP TIME: 15 MINUTES

This salad contains phytonutrients from across the spectrum. Red cherries and beets, white fennel, brown walnuts, mandarin oranges, and, of course, salad greens all help decrease inflammation, and the synergistic effects are more effective than one phytonutrient alone. Enjoy this colorful salad as a side, or add a serving of tofu or chicken to make it a meal.

2 tablespoons extra-virgin olive oil

3 tablespoons orange muscat champagne vinegar

¼ teaspoon turmeric

Salt

Freshly ground black pepper

4 cups mixed greens

1 fennel bulb, thinly shaved

4 mandarin oranges, peeled and sectioned (any seeds removed)

1 (8-ounce) package roasted beets, cut into wedges

¼ cup dried tart cherries, chopped

½ cup walnut halves

½ cup Parmesan cheese, shaved

1. In a large bowl, combine the olive oil, vinegar, turmeric, and salt and pepper to taste.

2. Add the greens, fennel, oranges, beets, cherries, walnuts, and Parmesan cheese and toss until evenly coated.

3. Serve and enjoy.

SUBSTITUTION TIP: You can omit the Parmesan cheese if you are eating dairy-free.

Per serving: Calories: 250/Total fat: 14g/Carbohydrates: 32g/Fiber: 7g/Protein: 7g

Classic Caesar Salad

CALCIUM-RICH | OMEGA-3 DHA AND EPA RICH | MONOUNSATURATED FAT | FIBER

SERVES 4 | PREP TIME: 10 MINUTES

This is a recipe I got from a friend who is known for his delicious Caesar salads. It is loaded with omega-3 DHA and EPA from the anchovies, as well as vitamin C and phytonutrients. This salad can easily be a main—just add extra anchovies or 2 ounces of grilled chicken.

1 egg

2 slices whole-grain bread

6 anchovy fillets, packed in oil, drained

1 large garlic clove

2 teaspoons Dijon mustard

1 teaspoon Worcestershire sauce

1 tablespoon lemon juice

¼ cup extra-virgin olive oil

4 cups romaine, chopped

2 cups kale, chopped

½ cup shredded Parmesan cheese

½ teaspoon freshly ground black pepper

1. In a small bowl, pour boiling water over the egg (still in the shell) and leave for 1 minute to coddle. Remove the egg with a spatula and set aside.

2. Toast the whole-grain bread and cut into cubes to make croutons. You can use whole-wheat or gluten-free croutons if you have them.

3. In a large bowl, combine the anchovy fillets and garlic. Using two forks or a muddler, mash into a paste.

4. Peel the coddled egg and remove the yolk; discard the white. Add the yolk, mustard, and Worcestershire sauce to the paste and whisk. Add the lemon juice and whisk together until it is well blended. Continue to whisk while you slowly add the olive oil. You can have someone help you add the oil if you have trouble keeping steady.

5. Toss the toasted croutons into the dressing, then add the romaine, kale, Parmesan cheese, and pepper. Toss lightly—just enough to coat the salad leaves.

6. Serve and enjoy immediately.

SUBSTITUTION TIP: You can use all kale, if you like, or all romaine. You can also use chopped Brussels sprouts for a crunch in place of croutons.

Per serving: Calories: 210/Total fat: 20g/Carbohydrates: 17g/Fiber: 4g/Protein: 10g

Shredded Brussels Sprouts Salad

DAIRY-FREE | GLUTEN-FREE | HEALTHY FAT | HIGH-FIBER | VEGAN

SERVES 4 TO 6 | PREP TIME: 10 MINUTES

Brussels sprouts are a superstar anti-inflammatory cruciferous vegetable. They have protective effects on our DNA, heart, digestive health, and detox pathways, which help defend against exposure to toxins. Make this hearty salad a meal by adding a quick protein such as canned chicken, salmon, or tuna.

4 cups Brussels sprouts

1 bunch Tuscan kale, stemmed and leaves chopped

1 avocado, chopped

½ cup chopped walnuts

¼ cup extra-virgin olive oil

2 tablespoons lemon juice

3 teaspoons red wine vinegar

1 small shallot, minced

2 garlic cloves, minced

¼ teaspoon turmeric

Salt

Freshly ground black pepper

1. With a sharp knife or mandoline, cut the Brussels sprouts into thin slices and put them in a large bowl.

2. Add the chopped kale, chopped avocado, and walnuts and toss to combine.

3. In a separate bowl, prepare the dressing by whisking together the olive oil, lemon juice, vinegar, shallot, garlic, and turmeric. Add salt and pepper to taste.

4. Drizzle the salad with the dressing and toss with salad tongs or two forks to combine.

MAKE IT EASY: You can purchase shredded Brussels sprouts and chopped kale to save prep time. You can also use ½ teaspoon dried shallot and 2 to 3 teaspoons minced garlic to eliminate mincing.

Per serving: Calories: 330/Total fat: 29g/Carbohydrates: 17g/Fiber: 8g/Protein: 7g

Grain Salad with Dried Plums

DAIRY-FREE | HEALTHY FAT | HIGH-FIBER | VEGAN

SERVES 4 | PREP TIME: 15 MINUTES | COOK TIME: 35 MINUTES, PLUS 30 MINUTES TO COOL

This fiber-packed, whole-grain salad is hearty enough to make a meal and is full of immune- and bone-health-supporting nutrients as well as powerful antioxidants.

3 cups water

1 cup farro (or other whole grain)

2 cups watercress, arugula, chard, spinach, or any combination

1 cup dried plums, chopped

½ cup walnuts

¼ cup mint, chopped

¼ cup basil, chopped

½ teaspoon salt

½ teaspoon pepper

¼ cup extra-virgin olive oil

2 tablespoons lemon juice

1. Combine the water and farro in a medium pot, bring to a boil, and simmer for 30 minutes, or until tender. Put the farro in a large bowl and refrigerate to cool before serving.

2. Once cooled, add the greens, dried plums, walnuts, herbs, and salt and pepper. Drizzle with oil and lemon juice, then toss to coat.

3. Serve and enjoy.

MAKE IT EASY: Batch cook your whole grains so you only have to make them once or twice per week. If the grains are leftovers, you will not need to wait for them to cool.

Per serving: Calories: 500/Total fat: 24g/Carbohydrates: 65g/Fiber: 9g/Protein: 11g

Bomb Diggity Dill Salmon Salad

DAIRY-FREE | GLUTEN-FREE | HEALTHY FAT | FIBER

SERVES 1 | PREP TIME: 10 MINUTES

This salad makes a great light meal. If you have Bomb Diggity Dill Dip on hand, prep time will only be 5 minutes. Smoked salmon is a no-cook way to get a tasty piece of fish, but be sure to read the label. The sodium per serving should be less than 20 percent of your daily value to keep sodium intake in check.

1 (3-ounce) package smoked salmon

1 cup arugula

½ cucumber, sliced

⅛ cup thinly sliced red onion

Salt

Freshly ground black pepper

3 tablespoons Bomb Diggity Dill Dip (page 83)

1. In a medium bowl, combine salmon, arugula, cucumber, onion, and salt and pepper to taste. Toss to mix ingredients.

2. Add the dill dip and toss the salad to coat.

SUBSTITUTION TIP: You can swap leftover baked salmon to cut the sodium down even further and keep this a speedy, no-cook meal. Alternatively, use canned tuna, salmon, or chicken.

Per serving: Calories: 160/Total fat: 5g/Carbohydrates: 4g/Fiber: 2g/Protein: 19g

Warm Kale Salad

GLUTEN-FREE | VEGETARIAN | HEALTHY FAT | HIGH-FIBER

SERVES 4 TO 8 | PREP TIME: 10 MINUTES | COOK TIME: 25 MINUTES

Sweet and savory flavors combine here to deliver a delicious and comforting kale salad. This hearty recipe makes 4 large salads, each big enough to be a meal, or you can serve 8 small salads as sides.

Salad

1 cup cooked quinoa

4 cups packed
  chopped kale

1 cup shredded carrots

½ cup low-sugar dried
  cranberries

1 cup walnuts

½ cup feta cheese,
  crumbled

Maple Dijon Dressing (makes 8 servings)

¾ cup extra-virgin olive oil

¼ cup maple syrup

¼ cup Dijon mustard

¼ cup apple cider vinegar

¼ teaspoon freshly ground
  black pepper

1. Prepare the quinoa according to package directions.

2. While the quinoa cooks, combine the kale, carrots, dried cranberries, walnuts, and feta cheese in a large salad bowl and set aside.

3. In a container with a lid, make the dressing by mixing the olive oil, syrup, mustard, vinegar, and pepper and set aside.

4. When the quinoa finishes cooking, toss it with the salad, which will warm the kale. Shake the dressing. Drizzle it over the salad, lightly toss again, and serve.

SUBSTITUTION TIP: You can swap the feta cheese for your favorite nut cheese or crumbled tofu. You will still get the creamy texture, and using tofu will provide some calcium, too.

Per large serving: Calories: 525/Total fat: 26g/Carbohydrates: 63g/Fiber: 12g/Protein: 16g

Make-Ahead Sesame-Soy Edamame Bowl

GLUTEN-FREE | VEGAN | HEALTHY FAT | HIGH-FIBER

SERVES 1 | PREP TIME: 5 TO 25 MINUTES | COOK TIME: 25 MINUTES

This recipe is for one, but I recommend filling a few to-go containers for the week. Batch cooking rice will cut down on future prep time, as using pre-cooked brown rice shaves the cook time down to zero. Sesame seeds are a source of monounsaturated fat and oleic acid, which promotes immune function and wound healing and decreases inflammation. They also contain calcium, iron, and magnesium.

⅓ cup brown rice

⅔ cup frozen, shelled edamame (thawed)

½ cup shredded carrots

1 cup cucumber spears

½ cup shredded cabbage

½ red bell pepper, sliced

1 tablespoon sesame seeds

1 tablespoon Szechuan sauce

1 teaspoon water

½ teaspoon ginger, freshly grated

1. Make the rice according to package instructions. This can be done ahead and cooled in the refrigerator.

2. In a medium bowl—or storage container, if making ahead—combine the edamame, carrots, cucumber, cabbage, and bell pepper. Sprinkle sesame seeds over the top.

3. Mix the Szechuan sauce with the water and drizzle over the salad. Top with the ginger, toss lightly, and enjoy.

SUBSTITUTION TIP: If you don't have Szechuan sauce, you can drizzle your salad with 1 teaspoon olive oil, 1 teaspoon low-sodium soy sauce, and 1 teaspoon white or rice vinegar and sprinkle with black pepper, chili pepper, and garlic powder. If you have sesame oil, add ¼ teaspoon.

Per serving: Calories: 370/Total fat: 12g/Carbohydrates: 53g/Fiber: 13g/Protein: 16g

Black Bean Taco Salad

GLUTEN-FREE | HEALTHY FAT | HIGH-FIBER | VEGAN

SERVES 4 | PREP TIME: 10 MINUTES | COOK TIME: 0 TO 25 MINUTES

This recipe makes 4 large salads or up to 8 side salads. This meal will keep you feeling full while providing an excellent source of fiber, which helps support immune and brain health by promoting growth of gut bacteria. The bacteria produce nutrients, neurotransmitters, and signals to immune cells.

½ cup dry quinoa or 1 cup precooked

1 cup water

1 tablespoon taco seasoning

4 cups purple cabbage, shredded

1 can black beans, rinsed

1 tomato, diced

1 yellow bell pepper, diced

1 avocado, diced

½ small red onion, diced

½ cup Cilantro-Lime Dressing (store-bought or see page 185)

1. Cook the quinoa with the water according to the instructions on the package. Season the cooking water with taco seasoning. Cool the quinoa in the refrigerator when it's finished cooking.

2. In a large bowl, combine the cabbage, black beans, tomato, bell pepper, avocado, and onion. Cover and place in the refrigerator if the quinoa is still cooling.

3. Once the quinoa is cool, combine with the salad mixture, add the dressing, and toss lightly.

MAKE IT EASY: This salad can be pre-dressed and will remain crisp due to the thick cabbage leaves.

Per serving: Calories: 406/Total fat: 13g/Carbohydrates: 60g/Fiber: 13g/Protein: 16g

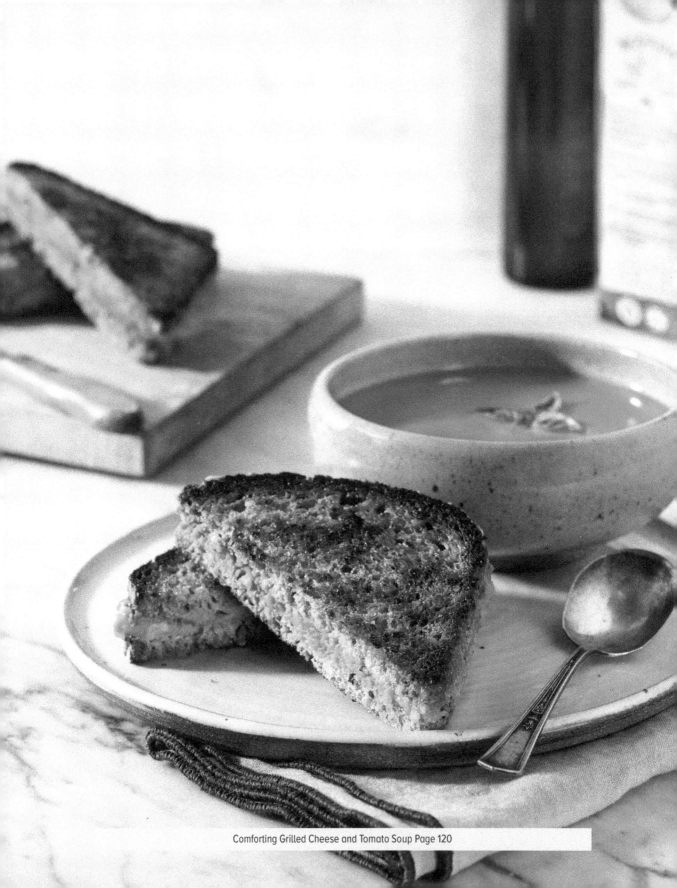

Comforting Grilled Cheese and Tomato Soup Page 120

CHAPTER EIGHT

Vegetarian Mains

Broccoli Macaroni "Alfredo"

GLUTEN-FREE | VEGAN | LOW-CALORIE | HIGH-FIBER

SERVES 4 | PREP TIME: 10 MINUTES | COOK TIME: 20 MINUTES

This recipe looks like a traditional creamy Alfredo dish, but it's made with cannellini beans and cauliflower. If you're cooking for picky eaters, this Alfredo sauce is a great way to sneak in some phytonutrient-rich vegetables and legumes.

1 head cauliflower

1 cup water

1 tablespoon avocado oil

½ small white onion, chopped

½ teaspoon garlic powder

1 (15-ounce) can cannellini beans, rinsed

½ cup nondairy milk

¼ teaspoon nutmeg

8 ounces chickpea pasta (or your favorite gluten-free pasta)

2 cups broccoli florets

1 tablespoon chopped fresh parsley

1. Remove the leaves from the cauliflower and cut the head into quarters. Separate the florets from the stem by running your knife between the florets and the thick core. Once the core is removed, you can break down any larger florets by giving them a quick chop.

2. Rinse the cauliflower. Place it in a large pot with the water. Simmer, covered, for about 20 minutes, then drain.

3. While the cauliflower steams, heat the avocado oil in a small sauté pan over medium heat. Sauté the onion with garlic powder for 5 minutes, or until soft and lightly browned.

4. When the cauliflower is soft and easily pierced with a fork, add the contents of the pot to a blender or food processor. Add the sautéed onions, rinsed beans, milk, and nutmeg, and blend until creamy. Add more milk if the consistency is thicker than desired.

5. Cook the pasta according to the package instructions.

6. Steam the broccoli florets in the microwave, covered, for 2 minutes.

7. Return the drained pasta to the large pot. Add the steamed broccoli and sauce and stir to combine.

8. Top with the chopped parsley and enjoy.

SUBSTITUTION TIP: Use roasted garlic cloves in place of garlic powder for a richer flavor.

Please use caution when blending hot liquids. Sometimes heat can cause pressure to build inside your blender or food processor.

Per serving: Calories: 379/Total fat: 9g/Carbohydrates: 59g/Fiber: 18g/Protein: 24g

Comforting Grilled Cheese and Tomato Soup

VEGETARIAN | HIGH-FIBER

SERVES 4 | PREP TIME: 5 MINUTES | COOK TIME: 10 MINUTES

This recipe is as comforting as a traditional grilled cheese with a boost of beta carotene from the sweet potato. The fat from the cheese increases your body's ability to absorb the beta carotene.

1 medium sweet potato

½ cup shredded mozzarella or cheddar cheese

8 slices whole-grain or gluten-free bread

1 tablespoon extra-virgin olive oil

1 package low-sodium tomato soup (for homemade, see page 95)

1 sprig fresh basil, stem removed, torn

Freshly ground black pepper

1. Pierce the sweet potato about four times with a fork or knife. Place it on a microwave-safe dish and microwave 4 to 6 minutes, or until soft.

2. Carefully remove the sweet potato from the microwave, allow it to cool, and then remove the skin.

3. In a medium bowl, mash the sweet potato with a fork, potato masher, or hand mixer. Once the potato is mashed to your preference, add the cheese, and stir to combine.

4. Spread the potato blend over four slices of bread, then top with the four remaining slices.

5. Coat a sauté pan or griddle with the oil and cook the sandwiches over medium heat for about 4 minutes per side.

6. Meanwhile, heat the soup per package instructions.

7. Pour the soup evenly into 4 bowls and top with torn basil and pepper to taste. Serve with the sandwiches.

SUBSTITUTION TIP: Use your favorite tortilla to make it a quesadilla instead of a sandwich.

Per serving: Calories: 390/Total fat: 9g/Carbohydrates: 60g/Fiber: 6g/Protein: 17g

Easy Caprese Pasta Salad

GLUTEN-FREE OPTION | HEALTHY FAT | HIGH-PROTEIN | HIGH-FIBER | VEGETARIAN

SERVES 2 | PREP TIME: 10 MINUTES | COOK TIME: 10 MINUTES

Fresh mozzarella is lower in sodium than regular mozzarella and it has a beautifully creamy texture. This pasta salad provides 100 percent of the vitamin A, more than half of the calcium, and more than one-third of the iron you need for a day.

4 ounces small, whole-grain or gluten-free pasta (such as rotini or farfalle)

2 teaspoons extra-virgin olive oil, divided

2 teaspoons balsamic vinegar

¼ teaspoon oregano

¼ teaspoon garlic powder

4 ounces fresh mozzarella, cut into ½-inch cubes

2 cups spinach

1 cup cherry tomatoes, halved

¼ cup fresh basil leaves, chopped into thin strips

Freshly ground black pepper

1. Prepare the pasta according to package directions, drain, and rinse with cool water. Toss with 1 teaspoon olive oil to prevent sticking.

2. While the pasta is cooking, whisk the vinegar, remaining 1 teaspoon of oil, oregano, and garlic powder together in a small bowl.

3. In a large bowl, combine the pasta, mozzarella, spinach, tomatoes, and basil. Drizzle with the oil and vinegar mixture and toss to coat.

4. Finish with black pepper and enjoy.

NUTRITION TIP: Vitamin A helps balance immune cells, decreasing the inflammatory response.

Per serving: Calories: 432/Total fat: 18g/Carbohydrates: 48g/Fiber: 8g/Protein: 20g

Quick Black-Eyed Peas and Collards

GLUTEN-FREE | VEGAN | HEALTHY FAT | HIGH-FIBER

SERVES 3 | PREP TIME: 6 MINUTES | COOK TIME: 20 MINUTES

This spin on a Southern dish is made with two highly anti-inflammatory ingredients—black-eyed peas and collard greens—and also packs amazing cholesterol-lowering and detox-supporting properties. Rich in fiber, folate, manganese, and vitamin A, this recipe is also a good source of protein.

1 tablespoon extra-virgin olive oil

1 onion, finely chopped

3 garlic cloves, finely chopped

½ teaspoon smoked paprika

1 bunch collard greens (about 7 cups)

1 (15-ounce) can black-eyed peas, drained and rinsed

2 cups reduced-sodium vegetable stock

1. In a large pot, warm the oil over medium heat. Add the onion, garlic, and paprika. Sauté for 5 minutes, or until the onions are soft and fragrant.

2. Using your hands, remove the collard leaves from the thick stems. Tear the leaves into bite-size pieces or give them a quick chop.

3. Add the greens to the pan and stir, lightly sautéing. Add the black-eyed peas and vegetable stock and bring to a boil.

4. Reduce the heat and simmer for 15 minutes.

SERVING SUGGESTION: Serve with a side of corn bread or top with corn bread croutons.

Per serving: Calories: 212/Total fat: 7g/Carbohydrates: 29g/Fiber: 7g/Protein: 13g

Savory Lentil-Bruschetta Shrooms

GLUTEN-FREE | LOW-CALORIE | HIGH-FIBER | VEGETARIAN

SERVES 2 | PREP TIME: 10 MINUTES | COOK TIME: 20 MINUTES

Lentils are loaded with fiber, protein, and nutrients; however, they can take a long time to cook, depending on how old they are. Fortunately, you can buy precooked lentils to save time. Feel free to use dried lentils if you prefer.

4 portobello mushrooms

4 teaspoons balsamic vinegar

Freshly ground black pepper

1 tablespoon extra-virgin olive oil

2 garlic cloves, chopped

½ cup diced onion

5 leaves fresh sage, chopped

1 cup pre-steamed lentils

1 cup chopped tomatoes (I like cherry tomatoes for this)

2 ounces goat cheese crumbles

2 cups arugula

1. Preheat the oven or set your toaster oven to bake at 425°F. Rinse the mushrooms, remove the stems, and pat dry with a paper towel. Place on a baking sheet, then drizzle 1 teaspoon of vinegar in each mushroom cap. Sprinkle with pepper.

2. When the oven is heated, put mushrooms in and set a timer for 10 minutes.

3. Meanwhile, heat the oil in a large pan over medium heat and sauté the garlic, onion, and sage for 5 minutes, or until the onions are soft.

4. Add the lentils and tomatoes, stirring to combine. Add the goat cheese crumbles and cover to allow cheese to melt slightly.

5. After 10 minutes, remove the mushrooms from the oven. Stuff the mushrooms with the lentil filling—it's okay if they are very full.

6. Return the mushrooms to the oven for 5 to 6 more minutes.

7. Plate the finished mushrooms on a bed of arugula and enjoy.

SUBSTITUTION TIP: You can grill the mushrooms, use smaller mushrooms and have more mushrooms per serving, or use them as an appetizer.

Per serving: Calories: 375/Total fat: 5g/Carbohydrates: 40g/Fiber: 14g/Protein: 21g

Roasted Veggie Tacos

GLUTEN-FREE | HEALTHY FAT | HIGH-FIBER | VEGAN

SERVES 2 | PREP TIME: 6 MINUTES | COOK TIME: 20 MINUTES

These tacos can be made on the grill. If you are cooking for one, cut down the recipe and use a toaster oven. The bright acidity from the lime and cilantro complement the creamy savory refried beans perfectly. Add cotija cheese if you would like.

1 zucchini, chopped

1 red bell pepper, sliced

½ medium red onion, chopped

1 cup frozen corn kernels

2 tablespoons extra-virgin olive oil

1 tablespoon taco seasoning

¼ cup fresh cilantro, roughly chopped

½ cup shredded cabbage

1 tablespoon lime juice

⅔ (15-ounce) can vegetarian refried beans

6 corn tortillas

1 avocado, diced

1. Preheat the oven to 400°F.

2. Place the zucchini, bell pepper, onion, and corn on a rimmed baking sheet. Drizzle with olive oil, add the taco seasoning, and toss to coat everything. Roast for about 20 minutes.

3. While the vegetables roast, combine cilantro, cabbage, and lime juice. Toss lightly to coat.

4. Heat the refried beans in a small saucepan over medium-low heat, stirring occasionally.

5. Heat the tortillas in the warm oven for 3 minutes or microwave for 15 seconds.

6. Spread the beans over each tortilla, then load with roasted veggies and top with avocado and the cabbage mixture.

SERVING SUGGESTION: Use 1 tablespoon of your favorite low-sodium salsa or hot sauce on each taco.

Per serving: Calories: 410/Total fat: 10g/Carbohydrates: 68g/Fiber: 15g/Protein: 11g

Thai Tempeh Lettuce Wraps

GLUTEN-FREE | HIGH-PROTEIN | HIGH-FIBER

SERVES 2 | PREP TIME: 10 MINUTES | COOK TIME: 10 MINUTES

Tempeh is a minimally processed form of soy. It is fermented, which improves its digestibility, decreasing the risk of gastrointestinal symptoms. Increased digestibility also means better absorption of phytonutrients from the soy, such as flavonoids, phytosterols, phenolic acids, and proteins.

½ cup brown rice

1 cup light coconut milk

1 teaspoon extra-virgin olive oil

1 cup shredded carrots

1 cup sliced red bell pepper

1 cup diced snow peas

Red pepper flakes (optional)

1 (7-ounce) package tempeh

3 tablespoons Sesame-Ginger Sauce (page 186)

6 to 8 large romaine lettuce leaves

¼ cup peanuts, crushed or chopped

1. Prepare the rice according to package directions, but substitute light coconut milk for water.

2. Warm the oil in a medium skillet and add the carrot, bell pepper, and peas. Sauté for 5 minutes, or until fragrant. Add red pepper flakes to taste (if using).

3. Using your hands, crumble the tempeh into the skillet, stir well, and add the Sesame-Ginger Sauce.

4. Cook for a few more minutes and remove from heat. Let cool before adding to the lettuce.

5. Stuff each lettuce leaf with tempeh mixture and top with crushed peanuts.

6. Enjoy with a side of coconut rice.

SUBSTITUTION TIP: You can use any dried herbs and spices you like when sautéing the vegetables. Garlic powder, onion powder, ginger powder, and turmeric all go well with this recipe.

Per serving: Calories: 520/Total fat: 25g/Carbohydrates: 48g/Fiber: 8g/Protein: 21g

Lentil-Cranberry Stuffed Acorn Squash

GLUTEN-FREE | HIGH-PROTEIN | HIGH-FIBER | VEGETARIAN

SERVES 3 | PREP TIME: 10 TO 30 MINUTES | COOK TIME: 55 MINUTES

Cranberries are loaded with phytonutrients, but fresh cranberries are only available seasonally. I've paired them with winter squash here, as they are both in season at the same time. Eating as locally and seasonally as you can will mean your food is fresher and more nutrient-dense.

2 cups beluga lentils

3 cups water, divided

1 tablespoon chopped fresh rosemary, plus 1 sprig

1½ tablespoons chopped fresh sage, plus 1 sprig

3 acorn squash, halved

2 tablespoons extra-virgin olive oil, divided

½ teaspoon salt

½ teaspoon freshly ground black pepper, divided

1 medium yellow onion, chopped

3 large celery stalks, chopped

1½ cups fresh cranberries

¼ cup pecans, chopped

¾ cup crumbled feta cheese

1. Rinse and pick through the lentils. Soak the rinsed lentils in 1½ cups water with a sprig of rosemary and sage for 45 minutes.

2. Preheat oven to 400°F.

3. Scoop out seeds from the halved squash with a spoon (you can wash the seeds and roast them later once they have dried). Arrange the squash in a baking dish or on a sheet pan and lightly drizzle the flesh side with 1 tablespoon olive oil. Season with salt and ¼ teaspoon black pepper.

4. When the oven is heated, roast the squash for 35 minutes, or until tender. Time varies depending on the size of your squash. Use a fork to determine if it is tender.

5. While the squash is roasting, sauté the onion and celery with the remaining 1 tablespoon olive oil in a large pot with a fitted lid for 5 minutes, or until tender. Add the remaining ¼ teaspoon pepper, fresh chopped herbs, lentils, and cranberries along with 1½ cups water. If you would like to use stock or broth instead, choose a low-sodium variety.

6. Bring the lentil-cranberry mixture to a boil, then reduce the heat to low and cover. Simmer for about 35 minutes, stirring occasionally. If the lentils look dry, add more water. Cook until the water is absorbed by the lentils and the lentils are tender.

7. Stir the pecans into the mixture, then spoon into the squash halves. Top with feta cheese and bake for an additional 10 minutes.

SUBSTITUTION TIP: You can swap the feta cheese for your favorite nondairy cheese substitute. To save time, soak the lentils the night before or use precooked lentils.

Per serving: Calories: 555/Total fat: 21g/Carbohydrates: 82g/Fiber: 24g/Protein: 35g

Barbecue Tempeh Bowl

GLUTEN-FREE | HIGH-PROTEIN | HIGH-FIBER | VEGAN

SERVES 2 | PREP TIME: 6 MINUTES | COOK TIME: 30 MINUTES

Barbecue is a summer staple, but you can enjoy this dish year-round by roasting your vegetables or, if you prefer, grilling them instead.

2 cups broccoli florets

2 cups cubed sweet potato

1 tablespoon avocado oil

½ teaspoon smoked
    paprika, divided

1 cup shredded
    purple cabbage

2 tablespoons apple
    cider vinegar

½ cup gluten-free
    barbecue sauce

¼ cup water

1 package gluten-free
    tempeh, sliced

Salt

Freshly ground
    black pepper

1. Preheat the oven to 400°F.

2. Place the broccoli florets and sweet potato cubes on a baking sheet, then drizzle with oil and sprinkle with some of the smoked paprika. Roast for 30 minutes.

3. Meanwhile, combine the cabbage, remaining paprika, and vinegar in a medium bowl. Toss to coat and set aside.

4. Heat the barbecue sauce with the water in a medium saucepan over medium heat. When it starts to bubble, add the sliced tempeh and stir to coat. Reduce the heat to low, cover, and allow to heat through, stirring occasionally.

5. Once the vegetables are finished roasting, build your bowl with barbecue tempeh, cabbage, broccoli, and sweet potato. Finish with salt and pepper.

MAKE IT EASY: You can purchase precut broccoli florets and sweet potato and shredded cabbage to cut down prep time.

Per serving: Calories: 415/Total fat: 8g/Carbohydrates: 29g/Fiber: 12g/Protein: 23g

Chana Masala over Cauliflower "Rice"

GLUTEN-FREE | VEGAN | HIGH-PROTEIN | HIGH-FIBER

SERVES 3 | PREP TIME: 6 MINUTES | COOK TIME: 20 MINUTES

Chana masala is a classic Indian dish bursting with flavor and phytonutrients, and the chickpeas are an excellent vegetarian source of protein. Enjoy this as an entrée, or use it as a side or snack.

1 tablespoon ground coriander

1 teaspoon turmeric

½ to 1 teaspoon garam masala

1 teaspoon smoked paprika

1 tablespoon avocado oil

2 teaspoons cumin seeds

1 medium yellow onion, chopped

2 teaspoons grated ginger

3 garlic cloves, chopped

1½ cups tomato purée

1 (15-ounce) can chickpeas, rinsed and drained

3 cups riced cauliflower

3 tablespoons water

Fresh cilantro or parsley

1. In a small bowl, mix the coriander, turmeric, garam masala, and paprika.

2. In a small saucepan, heat the avocado oil over medium-low heat. Add the cumin seeds and sauté for 1 minute, or until fragrant. Add the onion, ginger, and garlic and sauté for about 2 minutes. Add the spice blend and tomato purée. Stir to combine, then cover and let simmer for 10 minutes.

3. Add the chickpeas, stir, cover, and allow to simmer for 10 more minutes.

4. Meanwhile, heat a medium pan over medium heat with the cauliflower and water. Cover and allow to steam for a few minutes.

5. Serve the chana masala over cauliflower rice and garnish with fresh cilantro or parsley.

SUBSTITUTION TIP: Serve over ⅓ cup brown rice to make a complete protein. This is more important for people following a vegan diet.

Per serving: Calories: 290/Total fat: 8g/Carbohydrates: 47g/Fiber: 13g/Protein: 12g

Rainbow Pinwheels

GLUTEN-FREE | LOW-FAT | LOW-CALORIE | VEGAN

SERVES 2 | PREP TIME: 10 MINUTES

The more colorful your meals are, the wider variety of anti-inflammatory phytonutrients you will be getting daily. This colorful lunch can also serve as an easy, no-cook appetizer.

4 tablespoons hummus

1 cup spinach

2 Flatout brand protein wraps, or wrap of your choice

½ yellow bell pepper, thinly sliced

½ cup cucumber, thinly sliced

1 medium tomato, finely diced

Freshly ground black pepper

1 tablespoon lemon zest

1. Spread the hummus and spinach evenly over each wrap. Top with the bell pepper, cucumber, and tomato, distributed evenly. Season with pepper and lemon zest.

2. Starting at one end, roll up the wrap jelly-roll style.

3. Slice each pinwheel into 1-inch-thick medallions. You can refrigerate prior to cutting to allow the roll to set and use toothpicks to hold each piece together.

SUBSTITUTION TIP: You can use your favorite tortilla or gluten-free wrap.

Per serving: Calories: 204/Total fat: 6g/Carbohydrates: 28g/Fiber: 13g/Protein: 6g

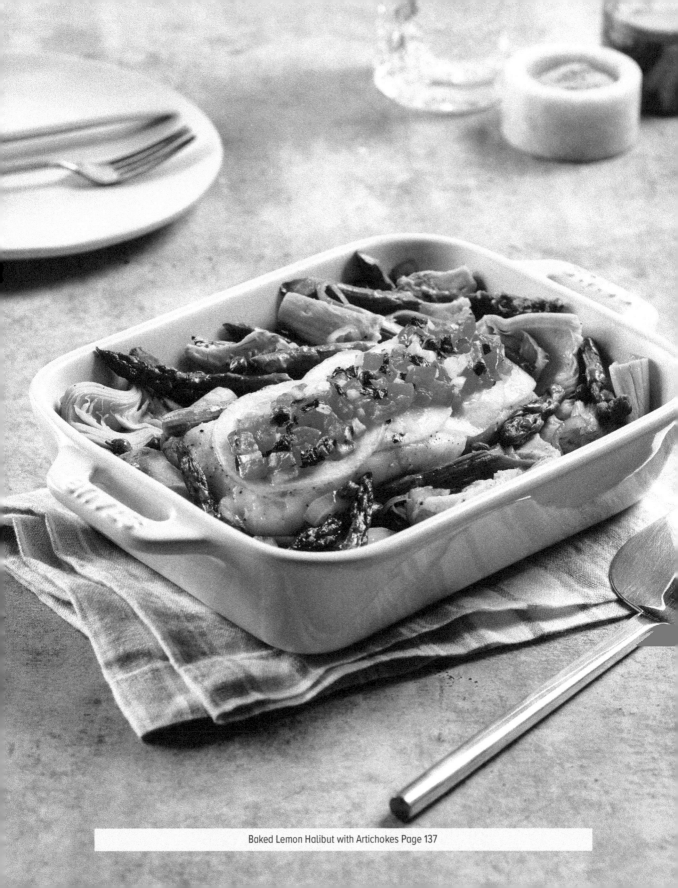

Baked Lemon Halibut with Artichokes Page 137

CHAPTER NINE

Seafood Mains

Classic Tuna Salad

GLUTEN-FREE OPTION | OMEGA-3 DHA AND EPA RICH | FIBER

SERVES 4 TO 8 | PREP TIME: 8 MINUTES

Tuna salad is a classic lunch or quick dinner. Children generally like it, too, which makes it a great introductory seafood for families trying to increase their intake of fish. The nutrition information listed is for a whole sandwich with two slices of whole-wheat bread. It will vary depending on whether a serving is a whole or half sandwich or includes any of the substitutions listed in the tip.

2 (5-ounce) cans tuna, albacore or light

2 celery stalks, finely diced

4 butter chip pickles, finely chopped

¼ small yellow onion, diced

½ cup mayonnaise made with olive oil

1 tablespoon yellow or Dijon mustard

Salt

Freshly ground black pepper

2 cups spinach

8 slices whole-wheat bread

1. Drain the tuna well.

2. Combine the drained tuna, celery, pickles, onion, mayonnaise, mustard, and salt and pepper to taste in a mixing bowl. Stir to combine well.

3. Serve over bread with spinach.

SUBSTITUTION TIP: You can use quartered bell peppers, quartered avocados, cucumber chips, or lettuce wraps in place of bread for your tuna salad. I recommend a combination of the options for variety.

Per serving: Calories: 380/Total fat: 14g/Carbohydrates: 37g/Fiber: 4g/Protein: 17g

Salmon Patties

DAIRY-FREE | OMEGA-3 DHA AND EPA RICH | GLUTEN-FREE OPTION | FIBER

SERVES 5 | PREP TIME: 8 MINUTES

Burgers are an American classic, but they don't provide any healthy EPA and DHA, which are essential fatty acids and building blocks for immune cells that decrease inflammation. Swapping salmon for ground beef is an easy way to eat familiar dishes while providing more variety and anti-inflammatory nutrients.

1 (14.75-ounce) can salmon, drained

¼ cup diced yellow onion

1 tablespoon chopped fresh dill or 1 teaspoon dried dill

½ cup plain bread crumbs, gluten-free

1 tablespoon fresh lemon juice

1 tablespoon Dijon mustard

2 large eggs, beaten

Kosher salt

Freshly ground black pepper

2 tablespoons extra-virgin olive oil

5 cups arugula

½ cup Bomb Diggity Dill Dip (page 83)

1. Drain the salmon well.

2. In a mixing bowl, combine the drained salmon, onion, dill, bread crumbs, lemon juice, mustard, and eggs. Mix well, then add salt and pepper to taste and mix one more time.

3. Form 5 equal patties. In a medium skillet, heat the olive oil over medium heat.

4. Cook the patties 3 to 4 minutes on each side. They should be golden brown.

5. While the patties are cooking, toss the arugula with Bomb Diggity Dill Dip. Serve the patties over the arugula.

MAKE-AHEAD TIP: These patties can be made ahead on a day you have more time. Store in an airtight container for up to 3 days.

Per serving: Calories: 280/Total fat: 11g/Carbohydrates: 12g/Fiber: 2g/Protein: 30g

Baked Fish and "Chips"

DAIRY-FREE | GLUTEN-FREE | HIGH-PROTEIN | LOW-CALORIE

SERVES 4 | PREP TIME: 6 MINUTES | COOK TIME: 20 MINUTES

This spin on a classic is baked instead of fried and uses green beans and sweet potatoes for the chips (aka fries). It's much more colorful and avoids the deep-fat frying of the traditional dish.

½ cup arrowroot powder
1 teaspoon garlic powder
1 teaspoon onion powder
¼ teaspoon paprika

2 sweet potatoes, cut into thin strips (like French fries)
1 egg
2 cups green beans

Salt
Freshly ground black pepper
2 or 3 (4-ounce) cod fillets

1. Preheat the oven to 400°F. Line a baking sheet with parchment paper.

2. In a small bowl, mix the arrowroot powder, garlic powder, onion powder, and paprika. Lightly coat the sweet potatoes with the mixture and arrange on the parchment paper.

3. Whisk the egg in a separate bowl. Dip the green beans into the egg, then dredge in the arrowroot mixture. Arrange on the baking sheet with the sweet potato.

4. Bake the vegetables for 20 minutes.

5. Meanwhile, salt and pepper both sides of the fish. Brush with the egg mix, then coat with the arrowroot mixture. Place in a baking dish. Once both fillets are coated, put them in the oven with the "chips" and bake for 15 minutes.

6. When everything is done, season with salt and pepper. Enjoy with organic ketchup or the dipping sauce of your choice. (Bomb Diggity Dill Dip [see page 83] works well.)

MAKE IT EASY: Use pre-breaded cod fillets. Check the ingredients if you're avoiding gluten and also look at the sodium—the daily value should be below 20 percent per serving to keep your sodium in check.

Per serving: Calories: 275/Total fat: 8g/Carbohydrates: 23g/Fiber: 3g/Protein: 32g

Baked Lemon Halibut
with Artichokes

DAIRY-FREE | OMEGA-3 DHA AND EPA RICH | GLUTEN-FREE | HIGH-FIBER

SERVES 2 | PREP TIME: 6 MINUTES | COOK TIME: 20 MINUTES

Halibut is a wonderful, lean white fish. Mild in flavor, it's a good choice for people just starting to eat fish. It's a great source of omega-3s, selenium, magnesium, and B vitamins, making it an excellent addition to an anti-inflammatory diet plan.

12 thin asparagus spears, ends discarded

1 cup frozen artichoke hearts, thawed

1 shallot, thinly sliced

1 tablespoon extra-virgin olive oil

¼ teaspoon oregano

Freshly ground black pepper

Salt

8 ounces halibut

¼ cup salsa fresca

4 lemon wheel slices

1 tablespoon capers

1. Preheat the oven to 400°F.

2. Cut or snap the asparagus spears into thirds. In a medium bowl, toss the asparagus, artichoke hearts, shallot, oil, and oregano and season with pepper. Arrange around the edges of a baking dish, leaving room in the middle for the fish.

3. Salt and pepper both sides of the halibut and place in center of the baking dish.

4. Spoon salsa over the fish and top with lemon wheels. Sprinkle capers over everything and bake for 15 minutes.

SUBSTITUTION TIP: You can use ¼ cup diced onions and sun-dried tomatoes if you don't have salsa fresca.

Per serving: Calories: 260/Total fat: 10g/Carbohydrates: 15g/Fiber: 5g/Protein: 27g

Sesame-Ginger Halibut and Mushrooms

DAIRY-FREE | GLUTEN-FREE | HIGH-PROTEIN | HIGH-FIBER

SERVES 2 | PREP TIME: 6 MINUTES | COOK TIME: 20 MINUTES

Mushrooms are a good source of fiber and nutrients such as selenium, a powerful antioxidant that promotes immune health. The sesame-ginger sauce pairs well with the cooked mushrooms, and the ginger provides healthy anti-inflammatory fat and anti-inflammatory compounds.

½ tablespoon garlic, grated

1 inch fresh ginger, peeled and grated

1 teaspoon fresh lemon juice

½ teaspoon lemon zest

3 thinly sliced scallions

1 tablespoon gluten-free low-sodium soy sauce

2 teaspoons sesame oil

1 teaspoon agave syrup

5 ounces sliced shiitake or cremini mushrooms, or both

Salt

Freshly ground black pepper

2 (6-ounce) skinless halibut fillets, or other white fish

¼ teaspoon chili flakes (optional)

4 cups spinach

2 tablespoons water

1 tablespoon sesame seeds

1. Preheat the oven to 400°F.

2. In a small bowl, whisk the garlic, ginger, lemon juice, lemon zest, scallions, soy sauce, sesame oil, and agave syrup. Set aside.

3. Lay out two pieces of parchment paper, about 9-by-13-inches. Distribute the sliced mushrooms on the lower third of the paper.

4. Salt and pepper both sides of the halibut and place it on top of the mushrooms.

5. Give your sesame-ginger glaze one last whisk and drizzle it evenly over both pieces of fish, reserving a bit. Top the fish with extra black pepper or chili flakes if you like a little spice.

6. Now make a pouch. Fold the parchment paper over the fish. Starting on one side, crimp the paper together, working your way around the entire pouch to make sure no liquid can escape.

7. Place the pouches on a baking sheet and bake for 12 to 15 minutes. While the fish bakes, heat a skillet over medium heat. Add the spinach, remaining sesame-ginger glaze, and water and quickly cover. Let the spinach wilt for about 30 seconds. Serve the fish over a bed of the lightly wilted sesame greens. Top with the sesame seeds.

MAKE IT EASY: You can store minced garlic and ginger in the freezer. This way, you always have some ready and you don't need to peel, chop, or grate anything.

Per serving: Calories: 250/Total fat: 5g/Carbohydrates: 25g/Fiber: 8g/Protein: 27g

Sea Bass and Scallop Ceviche

DAIRY-FREE | OMEGA-3 DHA AND EPA RICH | GLUTEN-FREE | FIBER

SERVES 6 | PREP TIME: 6 MINUTES | COOK TIME: 2 HOURS

For those times when you don't feel like cooking, this is the perfect make-ahead meal. It's a great summer lunch or dinner, as it does not require heat and is very refreshing. It also cooks in the refrigerator, so you don't need to keep an eye on it. You can leave the house, do laundry, or take a nap while it cooks.

½ pound sea bass
½ pound scallops (I like using large diver scallops, U-10)
½ cup lime juice
⅓ cup lemon juice

¼ cup orange juice
½ large red onion, chopped
2 jalapeños, chopped
1 cup grape tomatoes, chopped

⅓ cup fresh cilantro, chopped
1 small cucumber, chopped
1 small avocado, chopped
6 crispy tostadas

1. Using a very sharp knife, cut the sea bass and scallops into ¼- to-½-inch cubes. Put the cubes into a glass bowl or a serving bowl.

2. Pour the lime juice, lemon juice, and orange juice over the seafood.

3. Mix in the red onion and jalapeño, making sure the seafood is completely covered in citrus juice. If it is not fully covered, it will not cook evenly, so use extra juice if necessary.

4. Cover the mixture and place it in the refrigerator to cook—yes, cook!—for 2 hours.

5. Thirty minutes before it is done cooking, mix in the chopped tomatoes, cilantro, cucumber, and avocado. This will keep the colors beautiful and bright.

6. Serve over tostadas.

SUBSTITUTION TIP: No tostadas? No problem. You can use tortilla chips or crunchy vegetables as a vessel. Cucumbers, bell peppers, and hearty cabbage leaves work well.

Per serving: Calories: 390/Total fat: 17g/Carbohydrates: 40g/Fiber: 4g/Protein: 21g

One-Skillet Mediterranean Tuna

DAIRY-FREE | OMEGA-3 DHA AND EPA RICH | GLUTEN-FREE | HIGH-FIBER

SERVES 4 | PREP TIME: 6 MINUTES | COOK TIME: 20 MINUTES

Tuna can be a healthy source of protein. But if you are concerned about mercury contamination, stick with albacore and skipjack tuna, keep your portion sizes to 3 to 4 ounces per serving, and don't eat tuna more than once a week.

2 tablespoons extra-virgin olive oil

1 medium onion, diced

½ tablespoon minced garlic

4 anchovy fillets

2 medium yellow bell peppers, diced

2 medium green zucchini, spiralized (zoodles)

1 (28-ounce) can diced or crushed tomatoes

½ cup kalamata olives, sliced

1½ teaspoons dried basil

¼ teaspoon red pepper flakes

¼ teaspoon freshly ground black pepper

4 (3-ounce) tuna steaks

¼ bunch fresh parsley

1. Heat the olive oil in a large skillet over medium heat and cook the onion, garlic, and anchovy fillets for 5 minutes, or until the onions are soft and the anchovies have dissolved.

2. Add the bell pepper and zoodles to the skillet and sauté for 4 minutes, or until they are just slightly softened.

3. Add the tomatoes, sliced olives, basil, red pepper flakes, and black pepper. Stir to combine. Nestle the tuna down into the sauce, spoon some of the sauce over it, and cover with a lid. Simmer for 10 minutes, or until the tuna is white, indicating it is cooked through.

4. Remove the tuna and divide into 4 servings. Divide the zoodles into 4 bowls or dishes and serve topped with tuna and parsley.

SUBSTITUTION TIP: Serve over regular spaghetti to make this a heartier meal. If you are avoiding gluten, be sure the spaghetti is gluten-free.

Per serving: Calories: 290/Total fat: 8g/Carbohydrates: 30g/Fiber: 16g/Protein: 19g

Savory Sage Tuna with Baked Potato and Vegetables

DAIRY-FREE | GLUTEN-FREE | HIGH-PROTEIN | LOW-CALORIE

SERVES 4 | PREP TIME: 6 MINUTES | COOK TIME: 20 MINUTES

Tuna is a very lean fish, so it can become dry if overcooked. I recommend trying it medium-rare to rare. If you are not a fan of rare, start with medium and see how you like that. While tuna does provide omega-3s, keep in mind my advice about mercury: Eat only albacore or skipjack tuna in 3- to 4-ounce servings no more than once a week.

2 medium potatoes

1 pound tuna, cut into 4 pieces

3 tablespoons fresh lemon juice, divided

Salt

Freshly ground black pepper

2 tablespoons grated lemon peel

2 medium garlic cloves, pressed

¼ cup low-sodium vegetable broth

2 tablespoons fresh sage, minced

1 tablespoon fresh parsley, minced

Red pepper flakes

2 cups frozen vegetable medley

2 tablespoons butter

1. Pierce the potatoes with a fork and microwave for 5 to 6 minutes. Let the potatoes stand before cutting them in half.

2. Meanwhile, rub the tuna with 1 tablespoon fresh lemon juice and season both sides with salt and pepper.

3. Preheat a medium skillet over medium heat. Cook the tuna on each side for 1 to 2 minutes. Remove from the pan and set aside.

4. Keeping the pan over the heat, add the lemon peel, the remaining 2 tablespoons of lemon juice, garlic, broth, sage, parsley, and red pepper flakes to taste. Cook over medium heat for about 2 minutes.

5. Meanwhile, microwave the vegetable medley and plate ½ cup per plate. Top the vegetables with the tuna, place the potato with butter on the side, and pour the sauce over everything.

SUBSTITUTION TIP: Drizzle garlic- or sage-infused olive oil over the potatoes in place of butter.

Per serving: Calories: 275/Total fat: 8g/Carbohydrates: 23g/Fiber: 3g/Protein: 32g

Blackened Salmon Tacos

DAIRY-FREE | OMEGA-3 DHA AND EPA RICH | GLUTEN-FREE | HIGH-PROTEIN

SERVES 4 | PREP TIME: 6 MINUTES | COOK TIME: 10 MINUTES

This is one of my favorite meals. It's light but filling and loaded with colorful, phytonutrient-rich foods. It is also rich in healthy omega-3 fatty acids, which support a healthy immune system and decrease inflammation. There is a bit of sugar in this recipe, which helps get that crispy blackened crust on the salmon.

4 (4-ounce) salmon filets

2 teaspoons extra-virgin olive oil

8 small corn tortillas

Blackening Rub

1½ teaspoons paprika

1½ teaspoons cumin

1½ teaspoons dark brown sugar

½ teaspoon garlic powder

½ teaspoon onion powder

½ teaspoon kosher salt

½ teaspoon chili powder

¼ teaspoon black pepper

Slaw

2 cups broccoli slaw

2 cups shredded purple cabbage

1 tablespoon extra-virgin olive oil

3 tablespoons mayonnaise

2 tablespoons cilantro, chopped

2 small jalapeños, seeds removed and chopped

1 tablespoon lime juice

1. In a small bowl, combine and mix the paprika, cumin, brown sugar, garlic powder, onion powder, salt, chili powder, and black pepper. Sprinkle over the flesh side of the fish, reserving about 1 teaspoon for the slaw. (If you like a thick crust, you can double the blackening rub ingredients.)

2. Preheat a medium skillet over medium heat, add the olive oil, and coat the pan evenly.

3. Place the salmon in the preheated pan, flesh side down, and allow it to sizzle—don't flip it for 3 to 4 minutes, as you want it to char a bit. Flip it to the skin side and cover the pan for the last 4 minutes.

4. Meanwhile, combine the slaw ingredients in a large bowl and mix well.

5. Heat the corn tortillas. Fill each with about 2 ounces of salmon and at least ¼ cup slaw.

MAKE IT EASY: Just add a tablespoon of brown sugar to 1½ tablespoons of taco seasoning to make a quick blackening rub.

Per serving: Calories: 490/Total fat: 20g/Carbohydrates: 32g/Fiber: 4g/Protein: 32g

Almond-Pesto-Crusted Salmon

DAIRY-FREE | GLUTEN-FREE | HIGH-FIBER | HIGH-PROTEIN

SERVES 4 | PREP TIME: 5 MINUTES | COOK TIME: 15 MINUTES

Almonds add a nice crunch to delicate salmon, and the basil brightens up the dish and lends it a fresh, sweet, and savory component.

2 large zucchini, sliced

2 cups cauliflower florets

2 tablespoons extra-virgin
  olive oil, divided

Salt

Freshly ground
  black pepper

¼ teaspoon turmeric

12 ounces salmon

2 tablespoons pesto

2 tablespoons
  almonds, chopped

4 cups whole-grain
  spaghetti or other pasta

¼ cup sun-dried tomatoes

1. Preheat the oven to 400°F.

2. Arrange the zucchini slices and cauliflower florets in a single layer on a large baking sheet or dish. Drizzle with 1 tablespoon olive oil, salt and pepper to taste, then lightly toss with your hands. Sprinkle the turmeric over the cauliflower and lightly toss again.

3. In a separate baking dish, place the salmon skin-side down. Spread it with the pesto and top with chopped almonds.

4. Place the vegetables and salmon in the oven and bake for 15 to 18 minutes.

5. Meanwhile, prepare the spaghetti according to package directions. After draining, return to the pan to toss with the remaining 1 tablespoon of olive oil and sun-dried tomatoes.

6. Serve the salmon over the spaghetti with the roasted vegetables on the side.

SUBSTITUTION TIP: Spiralize the vegetables and replace the wheat pasta with chickpea, lentil, or other low-glycemic noodles.

Per serving: Calories: 385/Total fat: 11g/Carbohydrates: 45g/Fiber: 10g/Protein: 27g

Smoked Salmon Grain Bowl

DAIRY-FREE | GLUTEN-FREE | HIGH-PROTEIN | LOW-CALORIE

SERVES 1 | PREP TIME: 6 MINUTES | COOK TIME: 20 MINUTES

Smoked salmon offers the convenience of opening a pouch with ready-to-eat fish, rich in omega-3s. This is a perfect option when making a quick dinner for one.

½ cup cooked farro

¼ teaspoon garlic powder

¼ teaspoon onion powder

1 (3-ounce) pouch
  smoked salmon

2 tablespoons lemon juice

2 teaspoons extra-virgin
  olive oil

½ cup raw beets,
  thinly sliced

¼ fennel bulb, thinly sliced

2 tablespoons chopped
  fresh parsley

Salt

Freshly ground
  black pepper

1. Prepare farro according to instructions, and add garlic powder and onion powder to the cooking water.

2. Meanwhile, combine the salmon, lemon juice, and olive oil in a small bowl and toss to coat.

3. In a serving bowl, top the cooked farro with the beets, fennel, parsley, and salmon mixture. Add salt and pepper to taste.

MAKE IT EASY: Drizzle garlic- or tarragon-infused olive oil over precooked farro to cut out the cook time.

Per serving: Calories: 374/Total fat: 14g/Carbohydrates: 41g/Fiber: 5g/Protein: 26g

Grilled Cedar-Wrapped Salmon and Vegetables

DAIRY-FREE | GLUTEN-FREE | HIGH-PROTEIN | LOW-CALORIE

SERVES 1 | PREP TIME: 5 MINUTES | COOK TIME: 30 MINUTES

Cedar wraps lend the fish a delicious, smoky flavor and make grilling a breeze—the thin wraps require only about 5 minutes of soaking.

1 (4-ounce) salmon fillet

6 asparagus spears

1 carrot, thinly sliced

1 teaspoon extra-virgin
    olive oil

Salt

Freshly ground
    black pepper

1 teaspoon fresh or dried
    rosemary, sage, thyme, or
    tarragon

1 lemon wedge

¼ cup cooked brown rice

1. Preheat the grill. Soak the cedar wrap and twine for 5 minutes.

2. Place the salmon on the cedar wrap along with the asparagus and carrot and drizzle with oil. Sprinkle with salt, pepper, and herb(s). Squeeze the lemon wedge over the fish.

3. Wrap the fish and vegetables with the cedar wrap and tie closed with twine.

4. Cook on the grill for 15 minutes.

5. Serve with vegetables and a side of brown rice (nutrition information includes ¼ cup cooked brown rice).

SUBSTITUTION TIP: Drizzle garlic- or herb-infused olive oil over the salmon and vegetables for a different flavor profile.

Per serving: Calories: 490/Total fat: 16g/Carbohydrates: 44g/Fiber: 6g/Protein: 33g

Miso-Glazed Cod with Cucumber Salad

DAIRY-FREE | GLUTEN-FREE | HIGH-PROTEIN | LOW-CALORIE

SERVES 4 | PREP TIME: 6 MINUTES | COOK TIME: 20 MINUTES

Traditionally used in Japanese cuisine, miso is a great addition to your diet and a good source of probiotics. It also contains protein, several B vitamins, calcium, copper, zinc, magnesium, and iron. Since it keeps for up to 9 months, it's a great condiment to have on hand.

¼ cup white miso paste

¼ cup mirin

1 tablespoon sugar

½ teaspoon sesame oil

¼ cup rice wine vinegar or apple cider vinegar

1 teaspoon agave syrup or honey

¼ teaspoon red pepper flakes

2 cups cucumber, thinly sliced

¼ cup red onion, finely sliced

1 medium red bell pepper, finely diced

1 teaspoon sesame seeds

4 (4-ounce) cod fillets

3 scallions, thinly sliced

1. Preheat the oven to broil. In a small saucepan, cook the miso, mirin, and sugar over medium heat. Whisk until the sugar is dissolved. Remove from the heat and set aside.

2. While the miso sauce cools, whisk the sesame oil, vinegar, agave, and red pepper flakes in a small bowl to make the cucumber salad dressing, or shake the ingredients together in a jar with a lid.

3. Put the cucumber, red onion, bell pepper, and sesame seeds in a large bowl. Drizzle with the dressing and toss lightly. Cover and place in the refrigerator while you bake the cod.

4. Place the cod in a glass baking dish and brush with the cooled miso glaze. Cook under the broiler for 8 minutes.

5. Top with scallions and serve with the cucumber salad.

SUBSTITUTION TIP: If you don't have mirin, use rice wine vinegar with a tablespoon of sugar.

Per serving: Calories: 203/Total fat: 2g/Carbohydrates: 23g/Fiber: 2g/Protein: 21g

Creole Shrimp Kebabs

DAIRY-FREE | GLUTEN-FREE | HIGH-PROTEIN | LOW-CALORIE

SERVES 4 | PREP TIME: 6 MINUTES | COOK TIME: 20 MINUTES

This is a take on a Southern dish without the sauce. You can easily add stewed tomatoes to your rice and serve the kabob on top for a more classic version.

1 cup brown or wild rice (2 cups cooked)

1 cup kidney beans

2 tablespoons low-sodium creole seasoning, divided

1 pound medium shrimp, peeled and deveined

2 zucchini, cut into 1-inch chunks

1 medium onion, cut into 1-inch chunks

1 yellow bell pepper, cut into 1-inch chunks

1 pint cherry tomatoes

1. Soak the skewers if using wood and not metal. Heat the grill to medium-high.

2. Prepare the rice according to directions. Add the kidney beans and 1 tablespoon creole seasoning to the finished rice. Stir to combine.

3. Toss the shrimp in the remaining 1 tablespoon creole seasoning.

4. Skewer a variety of shrimp and vegetables on each skewer.

5. Grill for about 3 minutes per side.

6. Serve over the rice and bean blend.

NUTRITION TIP: Shrimp is a source of antioxidant and anti-inflammatory carotenoids that have been shown to support the nervous system and musculoskeletal system. It also provides some omega-3s.

Per serving: Calories: 309/Total fat: 8g/Carbohydrates: 40g/Fiber: 7g/Protein: 32g

Seared Scallops with Peas and Carrots

DAIRY-FREE | GLUTEN-FREE | LOW-CALORIE | HIGH-PROTEIN

SERVES 2 | PREP TIME: 8 MINUTES | COOK TIME: 15 MINUTES

Scallops are a sweet, rich-tasting seafood that pairs wonderfully with peas, mint, and butter. (Butter is okay to use, in moderation.) Scallops are rich in B_{12}, iodine, phosphorus, protein, selenium, choline, and zinc.

2 teaspoons avocado oil, divided

2 cups spiralized carrots

½ teaspoon onion powder

Red pepper flakes

2 tablespoons butter, divided, plus 1 teaspoon

2 cups shelled fresh or frozen peas

1 tablespoon chopped mint

6 large sea scallops (U-10 if available)

1 teaspoon grated lemon peel

Salt and black pepper

1. In a large skillet, heat 1 teaspoon of avocado oil. Add the spiralized carrots, onion powder, and red pepper flakes to taste and sauté for 10 minutes, or until the carrots are tender. Add 1 tablespoon of butter to the pan when finished just to melt and coat the carrots.

2. Meanwhile, simmer the peas in water in a medium saucepan over medium heat. Stir once or twice and cook 6 to 8 minutes, or until tender.

3. When the peas are soft, drain and return to the pan. Add the remaining 1 tablespoon of butter and the mint. Keep warm over low heat.

4. Season both sides of the scallops with the lemon peel, salt, and pepper.

5. In a small skillet, heat the remaining 1 teaspoon avocado oil, then add 1 teaspoon butter. When the butter starts to bubble, add the scallops. Cook on each side for 2 minutes, or until a brown crust starts to form.

6. Serve the scallops over the carrot spirals and peas.

SUBSTITUTION TIP: You can microwave frozen carrot spirals and frozen peas to make this a 10-minute dinner—5 minutes prep and 5 minutes cooking.

Per serving: Calories: 390/Total fat: 18g/Carbohydrates: 30g/Fiber: 9g/Protein: 26g

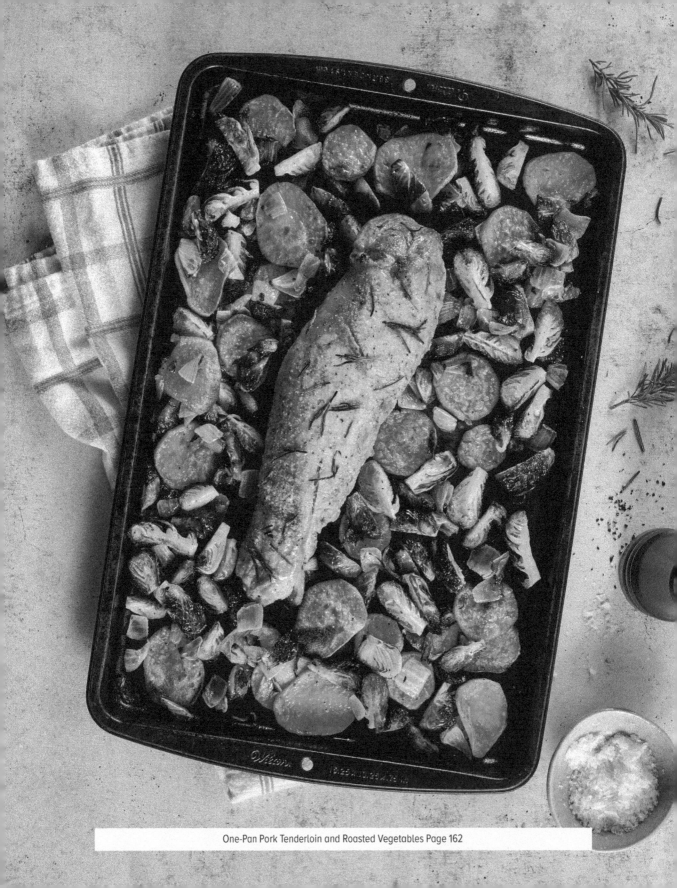

One-Pan Pork Tenderloin and Roasted Vegetables Page 162

CHAPTER TEN

Poultry and Meat Mains

Waldorf Chicken Salad Sandwich

DAIRY-FREE | GLUTEN-FREE | HEALTHY FAT | HIGH-FIBER

SERVES 5 | PREP TIME: 10 MINUTES

This classic, kid-friendly sandwich has a full variety of flavors, textures, colors, and food groups. It's a little sweet, a little sour, savory, creamy, and crunchy all at once. It is also easy to modify to accommodate food allergies and/or intolerances.

1 (12.5-ounce) can chicken
1 unpeeled apple, chopped
2 celery stalks, chopped
½ cup chopped walnuts

¼ cup dried cranberries
  or tart cherries, chopped
  (look for no sugar or
  reduced sugar)

¼ cup mayonnaise, made
  with olive oil
10 slices whole-grain bread
5 lettuce leaves

1. In a large bowl, combine the chicken, apple, celery, walnuts, cranberries, and mayonnaise

2. Mix well.

3. Spread over one slice of bread, then top with lettuce leaf and second slice of bread.

SUBSTITUTION TIP: You can replace the bread with cucumber boats or large cabbage leaves. Need it to be nut-free? Swap in pepitas for healthy fat and crunch.

Per serving: Calories: 410/Total fat: 18g/Carbohydrates: 50g/Fiber: 6g/Protein: 12g

Avocado-Chicken Pinwheels

GLUTEN-FREE | LOW-FAT | LOW-CALORIE

SERVES 4 | PREP TIME: 10 MINUTES

These pinwheels are rich and creamy, but don't worry—they're full of healthy monounsaturated fat from the avocado. They're also a great source of fiber, which promotes gut, immune, and brain health and can help with weight loss.

1 (12½-ounce) can chicken

1½ avocados, mashed

1 medium tomato,
  finely diced

½ small red onion,
  finely diced

½ orange bell pepper,
  finely diced

½ cup shaved cabbage

¼ cup shredded Mexican
  cheese blend

½ teaspoon cumin

½ teaspoon chili powder

½ teaspoon garlic powder

½ teaspoon paprika

Freshly ground
  black pepper

2 Flatout brand
  protein wraps

1. In a large bowl, combine the chicken, avocado, tomato, onion, bell pepper, cabbage, cheese, cumin, chili powder, garlic powder, and paprika. Season with pepper to taste.

2. Spread the mixture evenly over each wrap.

3. Starting at one end, roll up the wrap, jelly-roll style.

4. Slice the pinwheel into 1-inch-thick medallions. You can refrigerate prior to cutting to allow the roll to set and use toothpicks to hold each piece together.

SUBSTITUTION TIP: Omit the cheese if you are avoiding dairy.

Per serving: Calories: 326/Total fat: 16g/Carbohydrates: 20g/Fiber: 9g/Protein: 31g

Easy Chicken Sausage and Cucumber Salad

DAIRY-FREE | GLUTEN-FREE OPTION | FIBER

SERVES 1 | PREP TIME: 15 MINUTES | COOK TIME: 8 MINUTES

This meal is easy to throw together if you are feeling tired or too hot to cook a meal. Be careful, as not all sausage is equal: Look for organic and low-sodium sausage. If you choose a premade dressing, make sure it's also low in sodium and sugar.

1 low-sodium and low-saturated-fat chicken sausage link (Bilinski's is a brand I like)

1 cucumber, thinly sliced

1 medium tomato, chopped

¼ cup white beans

2 tablespoons feta cheese

1 tablespoon balsamic vinegar

1 teaspoon extra-virgin olive oil

⅛ teaspoon garlic powder

⅛ teaspoon onion powder

⅛ teaspoon dried oregano

Salt

Freshly ground black pepper

1. Cook the sausage in a toaster oven or in a small pan over medium heat for 5 to 8 minutes, or until lightly browned.

2. Meanwhile, combine the cucumber, tomato, beans, cheese, vinegar, oil, garlic powder, onion powder, oregano, and salt and pepper to taste in a medium bowl and toss to combine.

3. Cut the sausage into pieces and serve on top of the salad.

MAKE IT EASY: Use a premade dressing to cut prep time, or prepare homemade dressings in batches to allow for a quick meal.

Per serving: Calories: 236/Total fat: 6g/Carbohydrates: 25g/Fiber: 2g/Protein: 27g

Lemon-Turmeric Chicken Breast

DAIRY-FREE | GLUTEN-FREE | HEALTHY FAT | FIBER

SERVES 6 | PREP TIME: 15 MINUTES

This bright (colored and tasting) lemon-turmeric chicken is loaded with antioxidants that fight free radicals. Turmeric contains curcumin, the powerful anti-inflammatory compound that gives this chicken its bright hue. Purple sweet potatoes and green beans make this a fun, colorful meal.

2 tablespoons avocado oil

4 tablespoons lemon juice

1 teaspoon lemon zest

2 garlic cloves, minced

1 tablespoon turmeric

¼ teaspoon cumin

Salt

Freshly ground
    black pepper

1 pound chicken breast

2 cups purple potato, cut
    into ¼-inch medallions

2 cups green beans, rinsed
    and stems discarded

2 tablespoons extra-virgin
    olive oil

1 small onion, cut
    into wedges

1. Preheat the oven to 375°F.

2. In a small bowl, whisk together the avocado oil, lemon juice, lemon zest, garlic, turmeric, cumin, and salt and pepper to taste.

3. Place the chicken breast in a small baking dish, cover with the turmeric marinade, and marinate in the refrigerator for 30 to 45 minutes.

4. Place the potatoes and green beans in a separate baking dish. Drizzle with the olive oil and add salt and pepper to taste.

5. Add the onions to the chicken baking dish and bake alongside the vegetables for 25 minutes, or until the chicken reaches an internal temperature of 165°F. Flip the vegetables halfway through cooking.

SUBSTITUTION TIP: You can roast any vegetables for a side with the turmeric chicken, or serve the chicken in a green salad.

Per serving: Calories: 188/Total fat: 7g/Carbohydrates: 15g/Fiber: 2g/Protein: 16g

Whole Roasted Chicken

DAIRY-FREE | GLUTEN-FREE OPTION | PROTEIN

SERVES 6 | PREP TIME: 15 MINUTES | COOK TIME: 1 HOUR 15 MINUTES

Whole roasted chickens are very economical and provide a lean protein for 4 to 6 meals. Depending on the size of your chicken, you may need to adjust the cooking time.

1 whole chicken (about 3 pounds), giblets removed

Salt

Freshly ground black pepper

1 tablespoon onion powder

3 tablespoons butter, divided

2 garlic cloves, smashed

1 celery stalk, cut into 3 to 4 pieces

1 tablespoon extra-virgin olive oil

1. Preheat the oven to 400°F.

2. Place the chicken on a roasting pan, and season with salt, pepper, and onion powder inside and out. You can mix these ahead to avoid having to wash your hands between each seasoning.

3. Place 2 tablespoons of butter inside the cavity along with the crushed garlic cloves and celery pieces. Cut the remaining 1 tablespoon of butter into pieces and arrange on the outside of the chicken. Drizzle with olive oil.

4. Bake uncovered for 1 hour and 15 minutes or until the chicken reaches an internal temperature of 180°F.

5. Remove from the heat and baste using the drippings. Cover with aluminum foil and allow to rest for 30 minutes before cutting to serve.

SUBSTITUTION TIP: You can use rosemary or the herbs of your choice to season the outside of the chicken.

Per serving: Calories: 250/Total fat: 14g/Carbohydrates: 32g/Fiber: 7g/Protein: 7g

Slow-Cooker Turkey and White Bean Chili

GLUTEN-FREE | LOW-FAT | LOW-CALORIE

SERVES 12 | PREP TIME: 10 MINUTES | COOK TIME: 4 TO 8 HOURS

Slow cookers can save time on getting dinner ready while also making it easier to batch cook a meal. This slightly spiced chili makes 12 servings, so you can even freeze half and have ready-made meals.

1 teaspoon extra-virgin olive oil

1 large onion, chopped

3 or 4 garlic cloves, chopped

3 pounds lean ground turkey

4 (15½-ounce) cans cannellini beans, divided

1½ cups low-sodium chicken broth, divided

1 (14½-ounce) can diced green chiles

1 teaspoon cumin

1 teaspoon paprika

1 teaspoon chili powder (or more if you like spicy)

½ teaspoon salt

½ teaspoon oregano

½ cup plain Greek yogurt

1 avocado, sliced

1 bunch cilantro, chopped

1 jalapeño, sliced (optional)

1. Heat the oil in a large skillet over medium heat. Put the onions and garlic in the pan and sauté for 3 minutes.

2. Add the turkey and cook, breaking it apart, for 8 to 10 minutes, or until it is no longer pink.

3. Meanwhile, purée 1 can of cannellini beans and 1 cup of the broth in a blender or food processor. Pour into the slow cooker along with the remaining beans, broth, green chiles, and spices.

4. Transfer the turkey mixture to the slow cooker and cook on low for 8 hours or high for 4 hours.

5. Stir in the Greek yogurt and cook for an additional 3 to 5 minutes.

6. Top with sliced avocado, cilantro, and jalapeño, if using.

STORAGE TIP: You can store precooked chili in the freezer for up to 3 months.

Per serving (without topping): Calories: 315/Total fat: 10g/Carbohydrates: 24g/Fiber: 8g/Protein: 31g

Savory Sage Turkey Meatballs

DAIRY-FREE | GLUTEN-FREE | HEALTHY FAT | FIBER

SERVES 4 TO 6 | PREP TIME: 15 MINUTES | COOK TIME: 25 MINUTES

Meal prepping and batch cooking make it easy to keep healthy options available. This recipe is the perfect make-ahead protein to create a meal in under 20 minutes and satisfy a craving for comfort food.

3 garlic cloves, chopped

¾ cup bread crumbs of your choice

1 teaspoon salt

1 teaspoon pepper

2 heaping tablespoons fresh sage, chopped

¾ large onion, chopped

2 eggs

2 pounds ground turkey

1. Preheat the oven to 350°F.

2. In a large bowl, combine the garlic, bread crumbs, salt, pepper, sage, and onion and mix.

3. Whisk the eggs and add with the turkey to the mixture.

4. Roll into 1- to 1½-inch balls (makes 30 meatballs).

5. Place the meatballs on lightly oiled baking sheets.

6. Bake for 25 minutes, flipping halfway through. The meatballs should be lightly browned and reach an internal temperature of 165°F.

7. Serve with sautéed spinach and mushrooms and your favorite spaghetti.

MAKE IT EASY: Thaw frozen meatballs in the refrigerator or the microwave for a quick thaw. Reheat in the oven at 300°F for 15 minutes or on the stovetop in the sauce of your choice for about 10 minutes.

Per serving: Calories: 439/Total fat: 20g/Carbohydrates: 18g/Fiber: 2g/Protein: 49g

Slow-Cooker Chicken Cassoulet

DAIRY-FREE | GLUTEN-FREE | HIGH-PROTEIN | HIGH-FIBER

SERVES 6 TO 8 | PREP TIME: 20 MINUTES | COOK TIME: 4 TO 8 HOURS

This is a lighter, easier version of the French dish, which is traditionally prepared with duck and sausage. With onions, garlic, celery, carrots, and tomatoes, it does not skimp on flavor or phytonutrients.

3 tablespoons extra-virgin olive oil

2 links natural chicken sausage, cut into 1-inch pieces (Bilinski's or Applegate brands are good, lower-sodium options)

1 pound chicken thighs (about 4)

1 pound chicken legs (4 to 6)

3 to 4 garlic cloves, minced

1 large onion, coarsely chopped

3 large carrots, cut into ½-inch slices

2 celery stalks, cut into ½-inch slices

2 (15-ounce) cans cannellini beans, drained and rinsed

1 (14.5-ounce) can diced tomatoes

¾ cups chicken broth

1 bunch of fresh herbs (parsley or thyme)

¼ teaspoon freshly ground black pepper

1. Heat the oil in a large sauté pan over medium heat and brown the sausage and chicken, a few pieces at a time, and set the seared pieces aside. This step is optional, but it adds more flavor to the dish.

2. Put the garlic, onion, carrots, and celery in the same pan and sauté for 3 minutes. Remove from heat.

3. Roughly chop the meat and put it in the slow cooker along with the vegetables, beans, tomatoes, chicken broth, herbs, and pepper. Stir to mix the flavors, then cook on low for 6 to 8 hours or high for 4 to 6 hours.

4. Serve with a simple side salad or enjoy on its own.

SUBSTITUTION TIP: You can use boneless chicken thighs or breasts to make cutting easier. Using chicken breast will also reduce the fat.

Per larger serving: Calories: 370/Total fat: 13g/Carbohydrates: 30g/Fiber: 11g/Protein: 35g

One-Pan Pork Tenderloin and Roasted Vegetables

DAIRY-FREE | GLUTEN-FREE OPTION | HEALTHY FAT | FIBER

SERVES 4 TO 6 | PREP TIME: 10 MINUTES | COOK TIME: 30 MINUTES

Pork tenderloin is a lean protein that has flavorful juices. I recommend a meat thermometer to measure when it is done. Lean meats can become dry when overcooked.

1 to 1½ pounds pork tenderloin

1 sweet potato, cut into thin wheels

2 cups Brussels sprouts, quartered

½ yellow onion, coarsely chopped

2 tablespoons extra-virgin olive oil

Salt

Freshly ground black pepper

1 tablespoon rosemary

½ teaspoon garlic powder

½ teaspoon onion powder

1. Preheat the oven to 450°F. Let the tenderloin sit out to come up in temperature.

2. Place the sweet potato, Brussels sprouts, and onion on a large baking sheet in a single layer. Drizzle with olive oil and season with salt and pepper to taste. Bake for 12 minutes.

3. Meanwhile, season all sides of the tenderloin with rosemary, garlic powder, onion powder, salt, and pepper.

4. After 12 minutes of baking, stir the vegetables and make room for the tenderloin on the baking sheet.

5. Bake the tenderloin and the vegetables together for about 15 minutes, flipping the tenderloin halfway through.

6. Measure the temperature of the tenderloin. It is done when the internal temperature reaches 140°F. Remove from the oven and allow to stand for 5 minutes before cutting.

7. Slice the pork into medallions about ¼ inch thick. Each serving should be about 4 to 5 medallions.

8. Serve with your favorite whole grain or beans for more fiber.

SUBSTITUTION TIP: You can use any vegetables you wish. Cut denser vegetables thin to ensure they cook fast enough. For example, beets and other root vegetables should be ¼ inch to ½ inch thick.

Per larger serving: Calories: 305/Total fat: 13g/Carbohydrates: 14g/Fiber: 3g/Protein: 32g

Slow-Cooker Carnitas

DAIRY-FREE | GLUTEN-FREE | HEALTHY FAT

SERVES 16 | PREP TIME: 10 MINUTES | COOK TIME: 4 TO 8 HOURS

Pork is a very good source of the B vitamin thiamin, which is important for energy production, immune health, and brain health. These flavorful carnitas are a delicious way to get about a quarter of your daily value of this important vitamin.

Carnitas

4 pounds boneless pork shoulder (or pork butt)

4 garlic cloves, minced

2 teaspoons salt

2 teaspoons freshly ground black pepper

2 teaspoons cumin

1 teaspoon chili powder

1 teaspoon dried oregano

¼ teaspoon cinnamon

Juice of 2 oranges

Juice of 1 lime

2 cups water

Tacos and Toppings

Corn tortillas, for serving

Radishes, sliced

Cabbage, shredded

Red onion, diced

Cilantro, chopped

1. Place the pork shoulder in the slow cooker. Rub with garlic, salt, pepper, cumin, chili powder, oregano, and cinnamon.

2. Combine the orange juice, lime juice, and water and add to the slow cooker. Cover and cook on low for 8 hours or on high for 4 hours.

3. Shred the meat in the slow cooker—it should be very tender and pull apart easily. Serve in corn tortillas topped with the radishes, cabbage, red onion, and cilantro.

SUBSTITUTION TIP: Skip the tortillas and make a carnitas bowl. Serve over brown rice and black beans. For crispy carnitas, place the shredded carnitas on a baking sheet under a preheated broiler for 5 to 10 minutes.

Per serving: Calories: 163/Total fat: 8g/Carbohydrates: 3g/Fiber: 1g/Protein: 20g

Grilled Marinated Tri-Tip

DAIRY-FREE | GLUTEN-FREE | HEALTHY FAT

SERVES 6 | PREP TIME: 20 MINUTES | COOK TIME: 20 MINUTES

Grilled tri-tip makes outstanding beef to top a green salad or for a beef sandwich. It is simple to prepare and allows variety for how you serve it, making it versatile for meal prepping.

1½ pounds tri-tip roast

2 garlic cloves, crushed

1 sprig rosemary, coarsely chopped

¼ cup red wine

¼ cup extra-virgin olive oil

1 teaspoon salt

1 teaspoon black pepper

1. Preheat the oven or grill to 450°F.

2. Combine all the ingredients in a zip-top bag, sealing the bag to minimize air. Gently shake to combine and coat the tri-tip evenly.

3. Marinate in the refrigerator for 15 to 20 minutes.

4. Place the tri-tip directly on the grill or on a roasting pan in the oven. Cook for about 20 minutes, or until desired internal temperature (140°F for medium rare, 145°F for medium). Turn the tri-tip during cooking every 5 to 8 minutes to cook on every side.

5. Place the tri-tip in aluminum foil to set after desired temperature is reached, then slice thinly. Serve with your favorite vegetables.

SUBSTITUTION TIP: You can use red wine vinegar or balsamic vinegar in place of wine.

Per serving: Calories: 245/Total fat: 15g/Carbohydrates: 1g/Fiber: 0g/Protein: 24g

50/50 Mushroom Burgers

DAIRY-FREE I GLUTEN-FREE I HIGH-PROTEIN I LOW-CARB

SERVES 6 I PREP TIME: 15 MINUTES I COOK TIME: 10 MINUTES

Mushrooms are a delicious pairing with beef because they are savory and have an umami flavor. Replacing meat with mushrooms also reduces calories, fat, and cholesterol while making a more environmentally sustainable burger.

14 ounces mushrooms

2 teaspoons Worcestershire sauce

2 teaspoons black pepper

2 teaspoons granulated garlic

2 teaspoons granulated onion

½ teaspoon salt

1 teaspoon paprika

1 teaspoon red pepper flakes (optional)

16 ounces lean ground beef (90%)

1. Wash the mushrooms and pat them dry with paper towels.

2. Pulse the mushrooms in a food processor with the Worcestershire sauce or chop very fine. Optionally, sauté or roast the mushrooms before chopping to bring out more mushroom flavor.

3. Mix the black pepper, granulated garlic, granulated onion, salt, paprika, and red pepper flakes (if using) to make the spice blend.

4. Mix the chopped mushrooms with the beef and seasonings.

5. Form into 6 patties.

6. Preheat a grill to 450°F and cook the patties for 6 to 8 minutes, flipping halfway through. Alternatively, bake the burgers on a sheet pan in a 400°F oven for 10 minutes, flipping halfway through. Serve on a bun or lettuce leaves with your favorite vegetable toppings and sauce.

STORAGE TIP: Uncooked, formed patties can be frozen for up to 1 month.

Per serving: Calories: 228/Total fat: 10g/Carbohydrates: 7g/Fiber: 2g/Protein: 26g

Lamb Kebabs with Mint-Yogurt Dip

GLUTEN-FREE | HEALTHY FAT

SERVES 5 TO 6 | PREP TIME: 15 MINUTES | COOK TIME: 20 MINUTES

Grass-fed lamb is a great source of protein, B_{12}, selenium, B_3, zinc, and phosphorus. Additionally, about half of the fat in lamb is monounsaturated, which is a heart-healthy fat. Lamb is popular in the Mediterranean diet, one of the healthiest ways to eat.

1 cup nonfat plain Greek yogurt

½ tablespoon mint leaves, chopped

¼ cup cucumber, peeled if waxed and finely chopped

2 tablespoons fresh lemon juice, divided

2 tablespoons extra-virgin olive oil

3 garlic cloves, crushed

¾ cup dry red wine

1 tablespoon rosemary, fresh or dried

Red pepper flakes

Salt

Freshly ground black pepper

1 pound lamb, cut into 1- to 2-inch cubes

½ cup zucchini, cut into 1-inch-thick slices

1 red onion, quartered

1 large red bell pepper, cut into 1- to 2-inch square chunks

1. In a medium bowl, combine the yogurt, mint, cucumber, and 1 tablespoon lemon juice. Stir to combine and store covered in the refrigerator.

2. In a large zip-top bag, combine the olive oil, remaining 1 tablespoon lemon juice, garlic, red wine, and rosemary and add red pepper flakes, salt, and pepper to taste. Place the bag in a large bowl to prevent leaking.

3. Put the cubed lamb in the bag with the marinade, seal while minimizing air in the bag, toss to combine, and marinate in the refrigerator for 15 to 20 minutes.

4. If using wooden skewers, soak them in water for at least 15 minutes before using on the grill.

CONTINUED

5. Meanwhile, preheat the grill, set to medium. If using the oven broiler, set it to high.

6. Design your kebabs, alternating different vegetables and lamb pieces on each skewer.

7. Cook for 15 to 20 minutes, turning the skewers every 5 minutes.

8. Enjoy with the yogurt dip and serve with a side of rice or whole-wheat pita bread.

SUBSTITUTION TIP: You can use beef or any other lean meat in place of lamb.

Per larger serving: Calories: 350/Total fat: 19g/Carbohydrates: 8g/Fiber: 1g/Protein: 23g

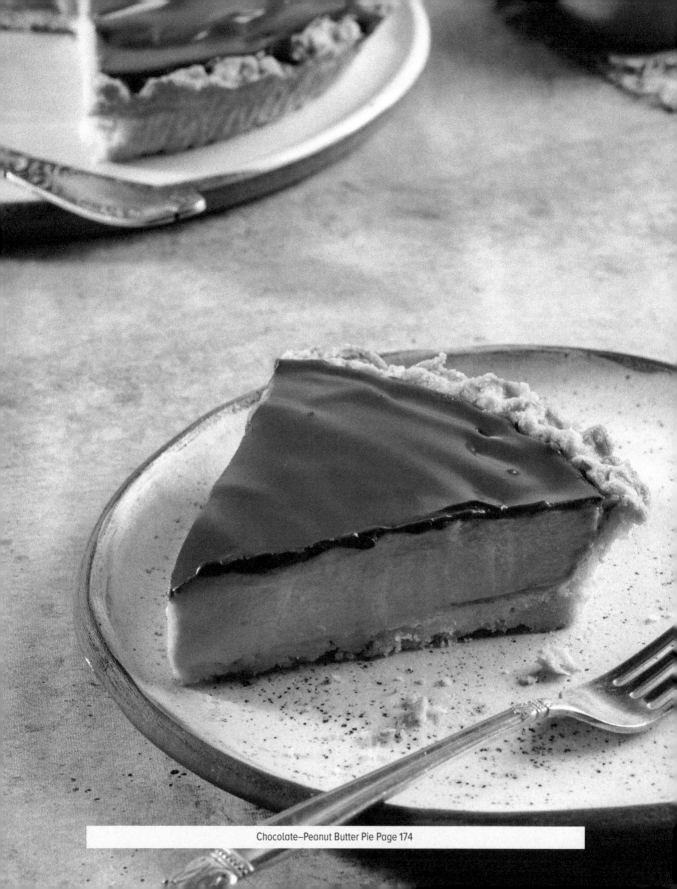

Chocolate–Peanut Butter Pie Page 174

CHAPTER ELEVEN

Desserts

Avocado and Key Lime Mousse Cups

DAIRY-FREE | GLUTEN-FREE | HEALTHY FAT | HIGH-FIBER

SERVES 8 | PREP TIME: 15 MINUTES | CHILL TIME: 20 MINUTES

Avocados make a great base for dessert because of their rich creamy texture. The bright-green color is perfect for a key lime dessert, too. Avocados are rich in nerve-protecting monounsaturated fatty acids and lutein.

⅔ cup unsweetened coconut flakes

⅔ cup walnuts

½ cup pitted dates

3 ripe avocados, pitted and peeled

3 ripe bananas, peeled

½ cup lemon juice

¼ cup lime juice

3 tablespoons lime zest

¼ cup organic raw honey

2 teaspoons vanilla extract

1. Combine the coconut, walnuts, and dates in a food processor or blender. Process or pulse until a crumb-like texture is achieved.

2. Remove from the processor and divide evenly in 8 small cups. (Using clear glass or plastic containers makes a pretty presentation.)

3. Add the avocado, banana, lemon juice, lime juice, lime zest, honey, and vanilla extract to the food processor or blender and blend until creamy and smooth.

4. Spoon the mixture over the crust in the cups. Place in the refrigerator to chill for 20 minutes before serving.

SERVING TIP: Top with a dollop of the whipped topping of your choice. Whipped cashew cream is an easy, 3-ingredient option. Just blend 1 cup raw unsalted cashews, ½ cup white grape juice, and 1 teaspoon vanilla extract.

NUTRITION TIP: You can experiment with decreasing the amount of honey. Start with 2 tablespoons and taste the key lime filling to see if it is sweet enough (4 tablespoons is the most you should use).

Per serving: Calories: 280/Total fat: 16g/Carbohydrates: 32g/Fiber: 7g/Protein: 4g

Sweet Lemon-Cherry Bean-Nut Dip

DAIRY-FREE | GLUTEN-FREE | HEALTHY FAT | FIBER

SERVES 8 | PREP TIME: 15 MINUTES | SOAK TIME: 1 HOUR TO OVERNIGHT

This dip has a texture like hummus, but it is a sweeter, richer experience, mimicking dessert. Cannellini beans make this dessert a healthy choice by providing fiber. They are also low-glycemic, meaning they do not impact blood sugar as much as other carbohydrates.

1 cup cashews

½ teaspoon vanilla extract

½ teaspoon vanilla powder, or additional teaspoon vanilla extract

3 tablespoons Meyer lemon juice

2 teaspoons lemon juice

1 tablespoon lemon zest

1 teaspoon honey

1 tablespoon almond or other milk

1 can cannellini beans, drained and rinsed

2 tablespoons dried tart cherries, chopped

1. Soak the cashews in water for 1 hour. (They can be soaked overnight as well.) Drain.

2. In a small bowl, combine the vanilla extract, vanilla powder, lemon juices, lemon zest, honey, and almond milk. Mix to combine.

3. Add the cashews, rinsed beans, and lemon-vanilla mix to a food processor or blender. Blend until smooth.

4. Transfer to a serving bowl or storage containers.

5. Top with chopped cherries—alternatively, stir them in.

6. Serve with apple slices, fruit chips, seed crackers, or other sweet crackers.

SUBSTITUTION TIP: Use the nuts and flavors of your choice. Soaked hazelnuts and cocoa powder would make a great bean-nut dip; just replace the lemon juice with almond milk.

Per serving: Calories: 150/Total fat: 8g/Carbohydrates: 16g/Fiber: 3g/Protein: 5g

Chocolate–Peanut Butter Pie

DAIRY-FREE | GLUTEN-FREE | HEALTHY FAT | FIBER

SERVES 8 | PREP TIME: 15 MINUTES | CHILL TIME: 3 HOURS

This is one of my absolute favorite desserts. It is dairy-free and gluten-free and can be made nut-free by swapping out the peanut butter for sunflower butter and using a nut-free pie crust. It is the perfect light, fluffy consistency, like a peanut butter mousse, topped with slightly firmer chocolate.

1 package silken tofu
1 cup creamy peanut butter
⅓ cup honey
1 teaspoon vanilla extract
¼ teaspoon salt

1 premade pie crust [I like using the crust from the Avocado and Key Lime Mousse Cups (see page 172)—just press in the bottom of a pie dish and set in the freezer for 1 hour]

8 ounces dark chocolate, finely chopped, or 1 cup mini semisweet chocolate morsels
⅔ cup nondairy milk (I like almond milk for this)

1. Drain the tofu of excess water by pressing with something like a cutting board. (Put the tofu on a paper towel on a cutting board. Place another cutting board on top and gently press the liquid out, draining it into a sink or dish drainer.)

2. Put the tofu, peanut butter, honey, vanilla, and salt in a food processor and blend until smooth and creamy. Use a spatula to scrape down the sides, ensuring it is mixed well. Pour the peanut butter mixture into a premade pie crust in a pie dish.

3. In a microwave-safe bowl, combine the chocolate and nondairy milk. Heat for about 60 seconds, or until fully melted. Stir to ensure it's mixed well.

4. Once the chocolate mixture is melted, pour it over the top of the pie. Set in the refrigerator for 3 hours or overnight.

MAKE IT EASY: Skip the crust and make chocolate–peanut butter squares instead. Simply pour the peanut butter mixture directly into an 8-by-8-inch baking dish, add the chocolate mixture per the recipe, and chill.

Per serving: Calories: 380/Total fat: 20g/Carbohydrates: 40g/Fiber: 4g/Protein: 11g

Black Bean Brownies

DAIRY-FREE | GLUTEN-FREE | LOW-FAT | FIBER | VEGAN

SERVES 10 | PREP TIME: 15 MINUTES | COOK TIME: 25 MINUTES

Ground flaxseed serves as a vegan egg in this recipe, and the black beans are the base of the brownies. This dessert packs healthy fat and fiber, unlike most sugar-laden brownies.

2 tablespoons ground flaxseed

6 tablespoons water

1 (15-ounce) can black beans, drained and rinsed

1 cup raw cocoa powder

½ cup coconut sugar

3 tablespoons avocado oil

2 teaspoons vanilla extract

1 teaspoon baking powder

1 teaspoon baking soda

$\frac{1}{16}$ teaspoon salt

1. Preheat the oven to 350°F.

2. Prepare the "flax egg" by mixing ground flaxseed and water. Let this sit for 5 minutes to form a gel.

3. Meanwhile, pulse the beans in a food processor and then scrape down the sides.

4. Add the flax egg, cocoa powder, coconut sugar, avocado oil, vanilla extract, baking powder, baking soda, and salt to the food processor and pulse well.

5. Pour the mixture into a lightly greased baking dish and bake for 25 to 30 minutes.

NUTRITION TIP: Add walnuts to make your brownie a filling snack. The walnuts will boost the protein and fiber, which will keep you feeling satisfied.

Per serving: Calories: 147/Total fat: 6g/Carbohydrates: 21g/Fiber: 3g/Protein: 4g

Spiced Banana-Oat Cookies

DAIRY-FREE | GLUTEN-FREE | LOW-CARB

SERVES 12 | PREP TIME: 10 MINUTES | COOK TIME: 20 MINUTES

These are not your traditional oatmeal cookies. There is no added sugar and no butter. The predominant fat in this cookie is monounsaturated fat—that's one smart cookie.

3 large, overripe bananas

1 egg

¼ cup extra-virgin olive oil

2 tablespoons spiced rum

1 cup old fashioned oats

¾ cup gluten-free flour (or all-purpose)

½ cup coconut flakes

½ cup chopped walnuts

1 teaspoon baking powder

1 teaspoon pumpkin pie spice

1. Preheat the oven to 350°F.

2. Mash the bananas, then combine them with the egg, olive oil, and rum in a large bowl. Pour mixture into a blender and mix well.

3. In a separate bowl, combine and mix the oats, flour, coconut flakes, walnuts, baking powder, and pumpkin pie spice.

4. Mix the dry ingredients into the wet mixture.

5. Drop the dough on a lightly greased baking sheet. Bake for 20 minutes.

SUBSTITUTION TIP: Make an "egg" with ground flaxseed and water. Combine 1 tablespoon ground flaxseed and 3 tablespoons water in a small bowl, and allow to gel for 5 minutes before using.

Per serving: Calories: 165/Total fat: 10g/Carbohydrates: 17g/Fiber: 2g/Protein: 3g

Chocolate-Coconut Truffles

DAIRY-FREE | GLUTEN-FREE | LOW-CARB

SERVES 15 | PREP TIME: 15 MINUTES

These truffles are a nice way to enjoy a little chocolate without all the added sugar that is in traditional truffles. A serving size is two truffles.

8 ounces dark chocolate (70 percent or more), finely chopped

½ cup full-fat canned coconut milk (unsweetened)

1 teaspoon vanilla extract (or your favorite extract, such as hazelnut, almond, orange, or coconut)

¼ cup cocoa powder or finely ground nuts

1. Place the chopped chocolate in a glass or metal bowl.

2. In a small saucepan, heat the coconut milk until it is simmering. Stir in the vanilla.

3. Pour the heated coconut milk over the chocolate and let it stand a few minutes to melt the chocolate. Stir the mixture until it is smooth and let it cool.

4. Place the cooled chocolate mix in the refrigerator for 30 minutes. Form the truffles by using a tablespoon to scoop rounds of the mixture and rolling it between your palms. Roll in cocoa powder or finely chopped nuts.

5. Place the truffles on a parchment paper–lined baking sheet and refrigerate overnight. These can be refrigerated in an airtight container for up to 1 week.

NUTRITION TIP: Chocolate is rich in antioxidants, such as catechins, which can help fight inflammation.

Per serving: Calories: 87/Total fat: 6g/Carbohydrates: 10g/Fiber: 1g/Protein: 4g

Mango-Strawberry Freeze

DAIRY-FREE | GLUTEN-FREE | LOW-CALORIE | FIBER | VEGAN

SERVES 4 | PREP TIME: 5 MINUTES

This is a creamier version of a fruit sorbet and is meant to be enjoyed right after making it. Mango is an excellent source of antioxidant vitamins A and C, as well as a good source of B vitamins and other important nutrients.

12 ounces frozen mango chunks

1 cup frozen strawberries

2 tablespoons nondairy milk

1. Combine the mango, strawberries, and milk in a food processor or blender.

2. Blend about 2 minutes, stopping to scrape the sides down and mix. Continue blending until smooth and creamy. Add additional liquid, if necessary, for a smooth texture.

3. Pour evenly into glasses and enjoy right away.

SUBSTITUTION TIP: You can use other fruit, but be sure to use a dense fruit such as mango, banana, or avocado to keep the creamy texture.

Per serving: Calories: 49/Total fat: 0g/Carbohydrates: 11g/Fiber: 2g/Protein: 4g

Chocolate Nice Cream

DAIRY-FREE | GLUTEN-FREE | LOW-FAT | FIBER | VEGAN

SERVES 2 | PREP TIME: 15 MINUTES

This creamy frozen treat can help cool you down and satisfy a sweet tooth without the dairy and loads of sugar that normally accompany ice cream.

3 bananas (should be ripe to overripe)

2 tablespoons almond milk

¼ cup unsweetened cocoa powder

1 teaspoon vanilla extract

2 teaspoons blackstrap molasses

1. Peel and slice the bananas, put them in a freezer-safe bag, and freeze.

2. Put the frozen banana slices in a blender or food processor with almond milk and blend.

3. Add the cocoa powder, vanilla, and molasses, and blend until smooth and creamy. (You may need to add an additional tablespoon of almond milk.)

4. Enjoy right away as soft serve, or pour into a container and freeze for an hour to scoop.

STORAGE TIP: If making ahead, Chocolate Nice Cream can be stored for a few weeks. However, if it has been frozen more than a few hours, let it sit out to soften before serving.

Per serving: Calories: 147/Total fat: 6g/Carbohydrates: 21g/Fiber: 3g/Protein: 4g

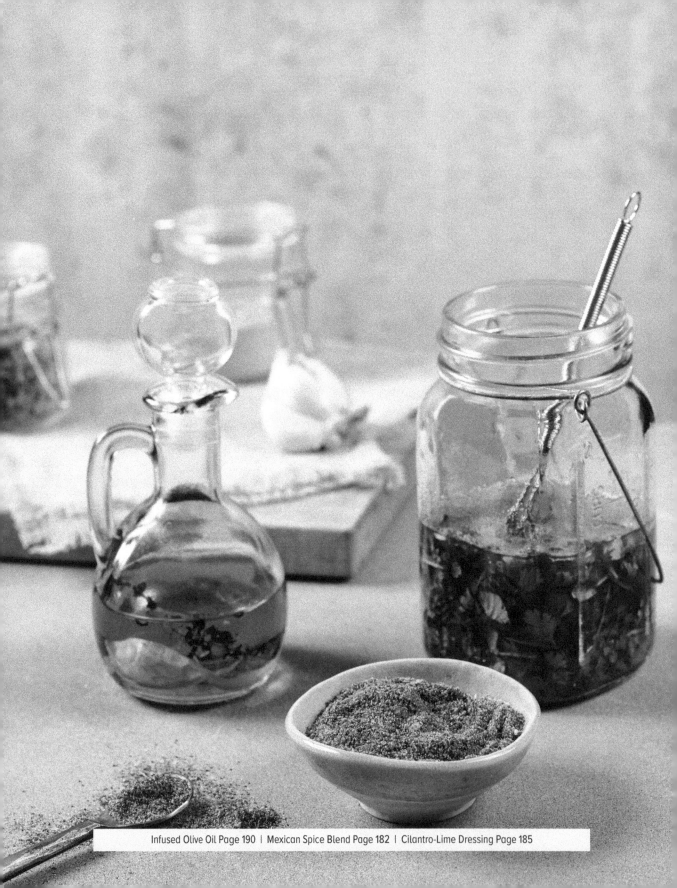

Infused Olive Oil Page 190 | Mexican Spice Blend Page 182 | Cilantro-Lime Dressing Page 185

CHAPTER TWELVE

Kitchen Staples

Mexican Spice Blend

DAIRY-FREE | GLUTEN-FREE | LOW SODIUM

MAKES ABOUT 9 TABLESPOONS | PREP TIME: 5 MINUTES

This simple spice combination can be used for any dishes you want to have a little spice or Mexican-inspired flavor.

2 tablespoons smoked paprika

2 tablespoons chili powder

2 tablespoons cumin

1 tablespoon garlic powder

1 tablespoon onion powder

2 teaspoons freshly ground black pepper

2 teaspoons salt

½ teaspoon dried oregano

1. In a small bowl, combine the paprika, chili powder, cumin, garlic powder, onion powder, pepper, salt, and oregano.

2. Store in an airtight container, preferably with a wide enough opening to fit a measuring spoon in it.

SUBSTITUTION TIP: Increase the amount of chili if you like it spicy. Use sweet Hungarian paprika for a less smoky flavor.

Per 1-tablespoon serving: Calories: 22/Total fat: 1g/Carbohydrates: 4g/Fiber: 2g/Protein: 1g

Italian Spice Blend

DAIRY-FREE | GLUTEN-FREE | LOW SODIUM

MAKES ABOUT 9 TABLESPOONS | PREP TIME: 5 MINUTES

The versatile Italian spice blend can be used to season vegetables before roasting or grilling, to season a salad dressed with just olive oil and vinegar, or in a marinade.

3 tablespoons
  dried oregano

2 tablespoons dried basil

2 tablespoons dried
  rosemary

2 tablespoons dried thyme

1. In a small bowl, combine the oregano, basil, rosemary, and thyme and mix well.

2. Keep the mixture in a small, airtight jar with a wide mouth.

SUBSTITUTION TIP: You can make a coarse Italian blend by using dried onion and garlic flakes instead of powder. The coarseness works well on meats to add texture.

Per 1-tablespoon serving: Calories: 12/Total fat: <1g/Carbohydrates: 3g/Fiber: 2g/Protein: <1g

Simple White Fish Blend

DAIRY-FREE | GLUTEN-FREE | LOW-SODIUM

MAKES ABOUT 5 TABLESPOONS | PREP TIME: 5 MINUTES

This blend can be used for salads and cooked vegetables, as well as for seasoning fish. The aromatic, slightly sweet flavor is fantastic on white fish, scallops, and shrimp. The turmeric brings a pop of color along with inflammatory-fighting phytonutrients.

3 tablespoons dried tarragon

1 tablespoon dried lemon peel

1 teaspoon freshly ground black pepper

½ teaspoon turmeric

1. In a bowl, combine the tarragon, lemon peel, pepper, and turmeric and stir thoroughly.

2. Store in a container that is airtight (small mason jars work well).

SUBSTITUTION TIP: You can use lemongrass or any citrus peel—lemon, lime, or orange. Dill pollen makes a great addition to this blend if you happen to come across it in the spice store. You can use it in place of or in addition to tarragon.

Per 1-tablespoon serving: Calories: 12/Total fat: <1g/Carbohydrates: 3g/Fiber: 1g/Protein: 1g

Cilantro-Lime Dressing

DAIRY-FREE | GLUTEN-FREE | LOW-SODIUM

MAKES ABOUT 1 CUP | PREP TIME: 5 MINUTES

One of my favorites, this bright and tangy dressing is perfect for salads, grain bowls, or dressing a taco. The fresh cilantro is loaded with anti-inflammatory and antimicrobial properties.

1 bunch cilantro, stems removed

½ cup extra-virgin olive oil

¼ cup lime juice

1 or 2 garlic cloves

2 teaspoons maple syrup or honey

¼ teaspoon onion powder

Salt

Freshly ground black pepper

1. Place all the cilantro, olive oil, lime juice, garlic, maple syrup, onion powder, and salt and pepper to taste in a blender and blend until creamy.

2. Keep refrigerated in an airtight container.

SUBSTITUTION TIP: Add one avocado to make a rich, creamy dressing.

Per ¼-cup serving: Calories: 259/Total fat: 27g/Carbohydrates: 5g/Fiber: 1g/Protein: 1g

Sesame-Ginger Sauce

DAIRY-FREE | GLUTEN-FREE | LOW-SODIUM

MAKES ABOUT 1 CUP | PREP TIME: 5 MINUTES

Sesame seeds are a source of anti-inflammatory and antioxidant fat, and they add texture to a dish. This sauce also has anti-inflammatory ginger, garlic, and citrus.

2 garlic cloves, minced

1 (1-inch) piece ginger root, peeled and minced

2 tablespoons sesame seeds

2 tablespoons light soy sauce

2 tablespoons honey

2 tablespoons fresh squeezed citrus juice (your choice)

¼ teaspoon toasted sesame oil

⅛ teaspoon cayenne pepper

1. In a small bowl, combine the garlic, ginger, sesame seeds, soy sauce, honey, citrus juice, sesame oil, and cayenne pepper and whisk to combine.

2. Store in the fridge in an airtight container.

SUBSTITUTION TIP: If you do not have fresh citrus juice, use rice vinegar or apple cider vinegar.

Per ¼-cup serving: Calories: 71/Total fat: 2g/Carbohydrates: 13g/Fiber: 1g/Protein: 2g

Asian-Inspired Stir-Fry Sauce

DAIRY-FREE | GLUTEN-FREE

MAKES ABOUT 1/2 CUP | PREP TIME: 5 MINUTES

This Asian-inspired stir-fry sauce will cut down the sodium compared to using prepared stir-fry sauces without sacrificing any flavor. Try adding chili, garlic, and onion powder for variation.

½ cup chicken or vegetable stock

2 tablespoons oyster sauce

1 tablespoon light soy sauce

1½ teaspoons fish sauce

1 teaspoon sugar

1. In a small bowl, combine the stock, oyster sauce, soy sauce, fish sauce, and sugar and mix until the sugar is dissolved.

2. Keep in the refrigerator in a sealed container.

MAKE IT EASY: Double up the recipe and store a batch in the freezer.

Per ¼-cup serving: Calories: 24/Total fat: 0g/Carbohydrates: 5g/Fiber: 0g/Protein: 1g

Orange Muscat Vinegar Dressing

DAIRY-FREE | GLUTEN-FREE | LOW-SODIUM

MAKES ABOUT 2 CUPS | PREP TIME: 5 MINUTES

This is a must-have dressing, as it goes well with so many different vegetables and fruits. I like pairing it with shaved fennel and beets, but it can be used on almost any salad.

1 cup extra-virgin olive oil

¾ cup orange
muscat vinegar

1 tablespoon dried tarragon

2 teaspoons freshly ground
black pepper

½ teaspoon salt

1. In a salad dressing jar with a lid, combine the olive oil, vinegar, tarragon, pepper, and salt.

2. Shake to combine, and be sure to shake again before using.

SUBSTITUTION TIP: If you can't find orange muscat vinegar, use white balsamic vinegar with 2 tablespoons of orange juice.

Per ¼-cup serving: Calories: 272/Total fat: 27g/Carbohydrates: 7g/Fiber: <1g/Protein: <1g

Simple Italian Dressing or Marinade

DAIRY-FREE | GLUTEN-FREE | LOW-SODIUM

MAKES ABOUT 1 AND 1/2 CUPS | PREP TIME: 5 MINUTES

This dressing doubles as a vegetable dressing or marinade. Most ingredients are pantry staples, so you should be able to whip this up almost anytime.

¾ cup extra-virgin olive oil

½ cup aged
   balsamic vinegar

2 tablespoons Italian Spice
   Blend (see page 183)

1 tablespoon lemon juice

1 teaspoon salt

1 teaspoon freshly ground
   black pepper

1. In a salad-dressing jar with a lid or another airtight container, combine the olive oil, vinegar, spice blend, lemon juice, salt, and pepper.

2. Shake to combine, and shake again before using.

MAKE IT EASY: You can use a preblended spice blend if you do not have the Italian Spice Blend made.

Per ¼-cup serving: Calories: 255/Total fat: 27g/Carbohydrates: 4g/Fiber: 1g/Protein: <1g

Infused Olive Oil

DAIRY-FREE | GLUTEN-FREE | LOW-SODIUM

MAKES ABOUT 1½ CUPS | PREP TIME: 5 MINUTES

Use infused oil to add flavor without extra sodium or sugar. For those with trouble digesting garlic, onion, or other highly fermentable foods, this will allow you to enjoy the flavor of those foods without the side effects.

¾ cup extra-virgin olive oil   1 bunch mixed herbs

1. Choose your flavor(s): chili flakes, rosemary, garlic, thyme, lemon peel, etc.

2. In a small saucepan, cook the oil and spice/herb of your choice over low heat for about 5 minutes, or until it reaches 180°F.

3. Remove from the heat and allow to cool to room temperature before transferring to your bottle. Seal and store in the refrigerator for up to 2 months.

SUBSTITUTION TIP: Use the citrus peel of your choice for a citrus-infused oil. This is great in salads and over cooked vegetables, to add acidity to a soup, or to drizzle over fruit.

Approximate calories per ¼-cup serving (will vary depending on the herbs): Calories: 243/ Total fat: 27g/Carbohydrates: 1g/Fiber: 1g/Protein: <1g

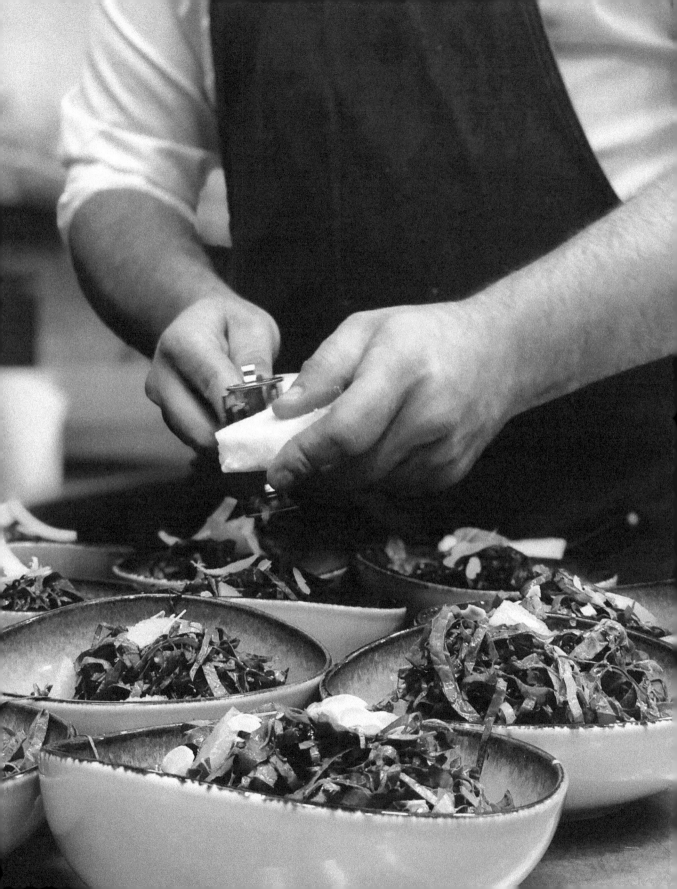

Tips for Going Out to Eat

Eating out can be difficult when you're trying to stick to a healthy diet pattern. It is important to socialize and have fun with friends, but you don't have to sabotage all the hard work you have put in to feeling better.

One thing you can do is plan ahead. Most restaurants have their menus online, and you can easily choose a few items in advance that fit your diet. When you're browsing the menu, be sure to look for foods that are baked, grilled, broiled, or steamed instead of fried. Avoid items listed as rich, creamy, or Alfredo—these are generally loaded with saturated fat. Look for entrées that have omega-3-rich fish such as salmon, trout, or tuna, especially if this is something you do not usually make at home. Check out the vegetarian options, which may be loaded with healthy vegetables, but be careful as some restaurants use a big plate of pasta as a vegetarian option.

Get comfortable asking your server questions about the menu. Ask if a poultry dish you are thinking about has the skin on it or if there is a vegetable you can substitute for a refined carbohydrate side such as macaroni salad. You may want to ask which dishes are gluten-free, dairy-free, or low in salt. If a cooking method is not listed, you can ask how the food is prepared. If you have allergies or food intolerances and you're uncomfortable explaining them, you can always call ahead and ask what they can prepare to accommodate your needs. Remember to ask for a to-go box as well—most restaurant portions are oversize, and overeating leads to blood-sugar spikes and dips, which leave you feeling tired.

One tip that I have recommended for those that have a hard time avoiding allergens in restaurants also works well for those trying to not stray from a healthy diet pattern. It may sound odd, but eat before you go. It's okay to order something light, like a salad, or abstain from eating at all, since the real reason you are going out is to socialize. If you're not hungry when you go out, you won't be tempted to have something that isn't good for you or makes you feel sick.

Desserts are difficult because there's no way to know how much sugar is in a prepared dessert. You can always ask for berries if you really want something, or convince the table to share dessert. (That way you can have just one bite.) Of course, you still have to be cautious of allergies and intolerances, and sometimes there is no good option. In that case, ordering a nice herbal tea is a good idea. It gives you something to enjoy while the rest of your group has dessert.

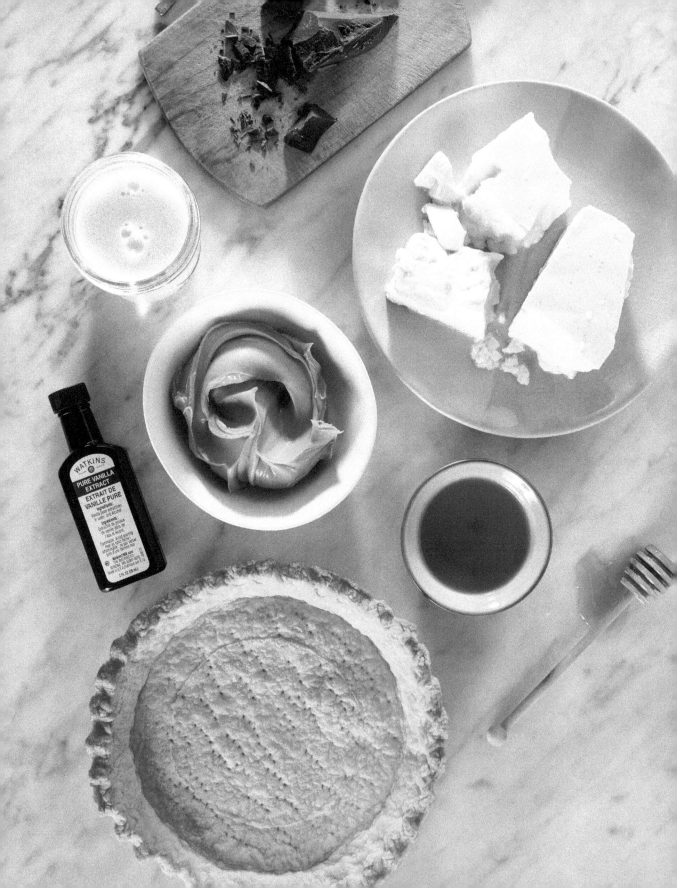

The Dirty Dozen and the Clean Fifteen™

A nonprofit environmental watchdog organization called Environmental Working Group (EWG) looks at data supplied by the US Department of Agriculture (USDA) and the Food and Drug Administration (FDA) about pesticide residues. Each year it compiles a list of the best and worst pesticide loads found in commercial crops. You can use these lists to decide which fruits and vegetables to buy organic to minimize your exposure to pesticides and which produce is considered safe enough to buy conventionally. This does not mean they are pesticide-free, though, so wash these fruits and vegetables thoroughly. The list is updated annually, and you can find it online at EWG.org/FoodNews.

DIRTY DOZEN™

1. strawberries
2. spinach
3. kale
4. nectarines
5. apples
6. grapes
7. peaches
8. cherries
9. pears
10. tomatoes
11. celery
12. potatoes

†Additionally, nearly three-quarters of hot pepper samples contained pesticide residues.

CLEAN FIFTEEN™

1. avocados
2. sweet corn
3. pineapples
4. sweet peas (frozen)
5. onions
6. papayas
7. eggplants
8. asparagus
9. kiwis
10. cabbages
11. cauliflower
12. cantaloupes
13. broccoli
14. mushrooms
15. honeydew melons

* A small amount of sweet corn, papaya, and summer squash sold in the United States is produced from genetically modified seeds. Buy organic varieties of these crops if you want to avoid genetically modified produce.

Measurement Conversions

	US STANDARD	US STANDARD (OUNCES)	METRIC (APPROXIMATE)
VOLUME EQUIVALENTS (LIQUID)	2 tablespoons	1 fl. oz.	30 mL
	¼ cup	2 fl. oz.	60 mL
	½ cup	4 fl. oz.	120 mL
	1 cup	8 fl. oz.	240 mL
	1½ cups	12 fl. oz.	355 mL
	2 cups or 1 pint	16 fl. oz.	475 mL
	4 cups or 1 quart	32 fl. oz.	1 L
	1 gallon	128 fl. oz.	4 L
VOLUME EQUIVALENTS (DRY)	⅛ teaspoon		0.5 mL
	¼ teaspoon		1 mL
	½ teaspoon		2 mL
	¾ teaspoon		4 mL
	1 teaspoon		5 mL
	1 tablespoon		15 mL
	¼ cup		59 mL
	⅓ cup		79 mL
	½ cup		118 mL
	⅔ cup		156 mL
	¾ cup		177 mL
	1 cup		235 mL
	2 cups or 1 pint		475 mL
	3 cups		700 mL
	4 cups or 1 quart		1 L
	½ gallon		2 L
	1 gallon		4 L
WEIGHT EQUIVALENTS	½ ounce		15 g
	1 ounce		30 g
	2 ounces		60 g
	4 ounces		115 g
	8 ounces		225 g
	12 ounces		340 g
	16 ounces or 1 pound		455 g

	FAHRENHEIT (F)	CELSIUS (C) (APPROXIMATE)
OVEN TEMPERATURES	250°F	120°F
	300°F	150°C
	325°F	180°C
	375°F	190°C
	400°F	200°C
	425°F	220°C
	450°F	230°C

References

Anderson, Per, and Mario Delgado. "Endogenous Anti-Inflammatory Neuropeptides and Pro-Resolving Lipid Mediators: A New Therapeutic Approach for Immune Disorders." *Journal of Cellular and Molecular Medicine* 12 (October 2008): 1830–47. doi:10.1111/j.1582-4934.2008.00387.

Efendi, Hüsnü. "Clinically Isolated Syndromes: Clinical Characteristics, Differential Diagnosis, and Management." Supplement, *Noro Psikiyatr Ars.* 52 (December 2015): S1–S11. doi:10.5152/npa.2015.12608.

Hewlings, Susan, and Douglas Kalman. "Curcumin: A Review of Its Effects on Human Health." *Foods* 6 (October 2017). doi:10.3390/foods6100092.

Kjølhede, Tue, et al. "Can Resistance Training Impact MRI Outcomes in Relapsing-Remitting Multiple Sclerosis?" *Multiple Sclerosis Journal* 24, no. 10 (September 2018): 1356–65. https://doi.org/10.1177/1352458517722645.

Mackay, Christopher P., Suzanne S. Kuys, and Sandra G. Brauer. "The Effect of Aerobic Exercise on Brain-Derived Neurotrophic Factor in People with Neurological Disorders: A Systematic Review and Meta-Analysis." *Neural Plasticity* 2017 (September 2017): 1–9. https://doi.org/10.1155/2017/4716197.

Martin, Clair R., Vadim Osadchiy, Amir Kalani, and Emeran Mayer. "The Brain-Gut-Microbiome Axis." *Cellular and Molecular Gastroenterology and Hepatology* 6 (April 2018): 133–48. doi:10.1016/j.jcmgh.2018.04.003.

Masjedi-Araani, Abass, and Roya Khanaliloo. "Comparison of the Efficacy of Cognitive-Behavioral Therapy (CBT) and Acceptance and Commitment Therapy (ACT) in Reducing Depression in Women with Multiple Sclerosis (MS)." *International Journal of Body, Mind and Culture* 5, no. 2 (April 2018): 112–21. http://ijbmc.org/index.php/ijbmc/article/view/117

Motl, Robert W., Dorothy Pekmezi, and Brooks C. Wingo. "Promotion of Physical Activity and Exercise in Multiple Sclerosis: Importance of Behavioral Science and Theory." *Multiple Sclerosis Journal— Experimental, Translational and Clinical* 4, no. 3 (July 2018). doi:10.1177/2055217318786745.

Phyo, Aung ZawZaw, et al. "The Efficacy of Psychological Interventions for Managing Fatigue in People with Multiple Sclerosis: A Systematic Review and Meta-Analysis." *Frontiers in Neurology* 9, no. 149 (April 2018). doi:10.3389/fneur.2018.00149.

Riccio, Paolo, and Rocco Rossano. "Diet, Gut Microbiota, and Vitamins D + A in Multiple Sclerosis." *Neurotherapeutics* 15 (January 2018): 75–91. doi:10.1007/s13311-017-0581-4.

Sanoobar, Meisam, Parvin Dehghan, Mohammad Khalili, Amirreza Azimi, and Fatemeh Seifar. "Coenzyme Q10 as a Treatment for Fatigue and Depression in Multiple Sclerosis Patients: A Double Blind Randomized Clinical Trial." *Nutritional Neuroscience* 19, no. 3 (2016): 138–43. doi:10.1179/1476830515Y.0000000002.

Simpson, Robert, et al. "Mindfulness Based Interventions in Multiple Sclerosis—A Systematic Review." *BMC Neurology* 14 (January 2014). doi:10.1186/1471-2377-14-15.

Strandwitz, Philip. "Neurotransmitter Modulation by the Gut Microbiota." *Brain Research* 1693 (August 2018): 128–33. doi:10.1016/j.brainres.2018.03.015.

Zostawa, Jacek, Jowita Adamczyk, Paweł Sowa, and Monika Adamczyk-Sowa. "The Influence of Sodium on Pathophysiology of Multiple Sclerosis." *Neurological Sciences* 38, no. 3 (January 2017): 389–98. doi:10.1007/s10072-016-2802-8.

Resources

Above MS (https://www.abovems.com/)

Change MS (https://www.changems.org/)

Multiple Sclerosis Association of America—Yoga and MS: Start Where You Are (https://www.mymsaa.org/videos/yoga-and-ms/)

National Multiple Sclerosis Society—Chapters (https://www.nationalmssociety.org/Chapters)

National Multiple Sclerosis Society—Exercise (https://www.nationalmssociety.org/Living-Well-With-MS/Diet-Exercise-Healthy-Behaviors/Exercise)

National Multiple Sclerosis Society—Resources and Support (https://www.nationalmssociety.org/Resources-Support)

Occupational Therapy Interventions for Multiple Sclerosis (https://www.multiplesclerosis.net/treatment/occupational-therapy-interventions/)

Resources on seafood and contamination (http://seafood.edf.org/tuna)

Index

Acknowledgments

Writing this book was more difficult than I imagined. I love cooking, educating about nutrition, and helping people make lifestyle changes, but writing a book that incorporates all of these was much different than I ever expected. I never could have completed this project without my best friend and love, Trent. He was very supportive during the process and helped me more than he knows.

A special thank you to Lacey Bromley and Susan Bennett for introducing me to exciting research and for supporting my growth as a registered dietitian. I am inspired by your passion to improve the lives of those you work with, as well as your drive to learn and expand the body of knowledge in the field of multiple sclerosis and neurologic disorders.

I am grateful for all my friends and family who have supported my nutrition-education journey and creativity in the kitchen. For those who have cooked with me—you know who you are—thanks for having fun with me in the kitchen.

Thank you to the entire Callisto publishing team that worked hard on this book as well. A special thank you to Michael and Mikki for your patience and for keeping me organized and on track.

About the Author

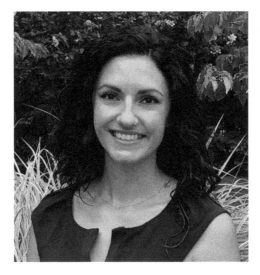

Noelle DeSantis received her bachelor's in nutrition from San Diego State University, where her passion for research started. She completed her dietetic internship and earned a master's in nutrition at the University at Buffalo, where her thesis was on diet manipulation and effects on various outcomes in people with multiple sclerosis compared to healthy controls. This was a randomized, cross-over design with a control group. She was inspired by the dedicated physical therapists she was working with, as well as the commitment of the participants in her study. She currently works for Buffalo Nutrition and Dietetics PLLC, offering one-on-one medical nutrition therapy at DENT Neurologic Institute. Noelle works with patients to develop individualized plans to help manage their symptoms and/or chronic disease. She also offers nutrition education as part of a holistic MS wellness program at Bennett Rehabilitation Institute.

CPSIA information can be obtained
at www.ICGtesting.com
Printed in the USA
BVHW011635140623
665820BV00001B/18

9 781641 528719